The Hatherleigh Guide

to

Managing
Depression

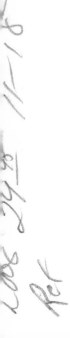

The Hatherleigh Guides series

The Hatherleigh Guide

to

Managing Depression

Hatherleigh Press • New York

Gary Holmes, PhD, CRC
Emporia State University (Emporia, KS)

John Homlish, PhD
The Menninger Clinic (Topeka, KS)

Sharon E. Robinson Kurpius, PhD
Arizona State University (Tempe, AZ)

Marilyn J. Lahiff, RN, CRRN, CIRS, CCM
Private practice (Englewood, FL)

Chow S. Lam, PhD
Illinois Institute of Chicago (Chicago, IL)

Paul Leung, PhD, CRC
University of Illinois at Urbana-Champaign (Champaign, IL)

Carl Malmquist, MD
University of Minnesota (Minneapolis, MN)

Robert J. McAllister, PhD
Taylor Manor Hospital (Ellicott City, MD)

Richard A. McCormick, PhD
Cleveland VA Medical Center-Brecksville Division (Cleveland, OH)

Thomas Miller, PhD, ABPP
University of Kentucky College of Medicine (Lexington, KY)

Jane E. Myers, PhD, CRC, NCC, NCGC, LPC
University of North Carolina-Greensboro (Greensboro, NC)

Don A. Olson, PhD
Rehabilitation Institute of Chicago (Chicago, IL)

William Pollack, PhD
McLean Hospital (Belmont, MA)

Keith M. Robinson, MD
University of Pennsylvania (Philadelphia, PA)

Susan R. Sabelli, CRC, LRC
Assumption College (Worcester, MA)

Gerald R. Schneck, PhD, CRC-SAC, NCC
Mankato State University (Mankato, MN)

George Silberschatz, PhD
University of California-San Fransisco (San Fransisco, CA)

David W. Smart, PhD
Brigham Young University (Provo, UT)

Julie F. Smart, PhD, CRC, NCC
Utah State University (Logan, UT)

Joseph Stano, PhD, CRC, LRC, NCC
Springfield College (Springfield, MA)

Anthony Storr, FRCP
Green College (Oxford, England)

Hans Strupp, PhD
Vanderbilt University (Nashville, TN)

Retta C. Trautman, CCMHC, LPCC
Private practice (Toledo, OH)

Patricia Vohs, RN, CRRN, CRC, CIRS, CCM
Private practice (Warminster, PA)

William J. Weikel, PhD, CCMHC, NCC
Morehead State University (Morehead, KY)

Nona Leigh Wilson, PhD
South Dakota State University (Brookings, SD)

The Hatherleigh Guide to Managing Depression

Project Editor: Joya Lonsdale
Indexer: Angela Washington-Blair, PhD
Cover Designer: Gary Szczecina
Cover photo: Christopher Flach, PhD

© 1996 Hatherleigh Press
A Division of The Hatherleigh Company, Ltd.
420 East 51st Street, New York, NY 10022

This book is printed on acid-free paper.

Compiled under the auspices of the editorial boards of *Directions in Mental Health Counseling, Directions in Clinical Psychology,* and *Directions in Rehabilitation Counseling.*

Library of Congress Cataloging-in-Publication Data

The Hatherleigh Guide to Managing Depression — 1st ed.
     p. cm. — (The Hatherleigh guides ; 3)
     Includes bibliographical references and indexes.
     ISBN 1-886330-10-7 (alk. paper)
     1. Depression, Mental. I. Hatherleigh Press. II. Series: The Hatherleigh guides to mental health practice series ; 3.
     RC456.H38 1995 vol. 3
     [RC537]
     616.85' 27 — dc20   96-33715
                                          CIP

First Edition: May 1996

10 9 8 7 6 5 4 3 2 1

About the photograph and the photographer

Prianon, 1994
A man looks out the window of his dark, depressing room into the hopeful, warm sunlight. The world outside his window offers limitless possibilities.

Christopher Flach, PhD, is a psychologist in private practice in southern California. An avid photographer for more than 20 years, his favorite subjects include people and nature. He has studied photography with Ansel Adams, and his work has been on display in public galleries and in private collections.

Table of Contents

Illustrations

Introduction

I have had a special interest in the problem of depression from the very beginning of my career in psychiatry. The first scientific paper I wrote, published in the *Archives of Neurology and Psychiatry* in 1954, was entitled "Intensive Psychotherapy in Depression." For 15 years, as director of the metabolic research unit at the Payne Whitney Clinic of The New York Hospital, I studied changes in calcium physiology associated with depression and was privileged to be among the first clinicians to use the new antidepressant medication called imipramine (Tofranil), which has become the gold standard of antidepressants.

In staff conference after staff conference, I listened to dozens of stories about the terribly stressful events that often precede the onset of depressive symptoms — divorce, the death of a loved one, business failure. I couldn't help thinking that many of these people seemed to have every right to be depressed. When I met my clients in sessions with their families, it often became apparent that family dynamics was a major source of their depression; without a change in clients' home environments, it would be difficult for many clients to recover and stay well. Early on, I could appreciate the complexity of depression, in which psychological, environmental, and biologic factors all played significant etiological roles.

In this context, I reformulated my own concept of what depression is — and what it is not. Being depressed, *per se*, is neither a weakness nor an illness. Rather, depression is the way healthy human beings respond to certain stresses, particularly those involving the loss of something meaningful to them. Depression can be viewed as an illness when it is not recognized and acknowledged, when it gets out of hand and overwhelms a client, when it persists, and — most important —

when the individual cannot recover from an episode on his or her own.

The Hatherleigh Guide to Managing Depression truly reflects this biopsychosocial model for the diagnosis and treatment of affective disorders. It offers a highly practical, hands-on approach for treating depression and contains many insights and perspectives required by any practitioner who intends to work with depressed clients or patients.

Peter Whybrow's excellent description of depressed clients points to several common maladaptive personality styles that stem from a failure to master the attachment-separation experience early in life, thus creating a special vulnerability to depression and an inability to manage it successfully. His insights set the stage for what Louis Jolyon West calls *integrative therapy*, the goals of which include promoting a patient's *functional wholeness* (a healing process); *existential continuity* (the integration of past experience with present and future coping); and *adaptive relevance* (a balanced, harmonious relationship with the physical, social, and moral environments).

Dr. West's suggestions about psychotherapy are echoed by Robert Howland, who, in discussing the treatment of dysthymia, advises an active and directive therapeutic stance, rather than a passive, uncommunicative one. He also stresses the importance of flexibility and cautions against therapists being too wedded to any particular theoretical model of treatment.

Vulnerability to depression can also be seen in people who hold powerful negative views about themselves, their worlds, and their futures. Robin B. Jarrett and A. John Rush address the faulty cognitions and perceptions that frequently underlie depression and describe how cognitive therapy can be an effective form of treatment for such cognitions. This approach goes beyond merely seeing cognitive therapy as a specialized technique and discovering ways to incorporate its principles in the context of general psychotherapy.

Patients with anorexia nervosa or bulimia nervosa have an extremely negative attitude toward themselves, with particular regard to eating problems and body image. As Arnold E.

Anderson demonstrates, depression is quite common in such patients. In anorexic patients, starvation induces depression. A depressive mood often initiates the dieting behavior, and weight gain can unmask an underlying depression. In a number of bulimic patients, the bulimic symptoms seem to regulate depressive symptoms.

Dr. Whybrow cites excessive dependence on a dominant person as an important maladaptive style in depressed clients. However, as John A. Birtchnell emphasizes, the therapist must distinguish between dependency as a long-standing personality trait requiring long-term therapy and dependency that can result from the immobilizing and self-diminishing effects of a depressed mood—a dependency that will usually subside with improvement and calls for tactful, empathic, reassuring management.

The first patient whom I treated for depression happened to be a very successful business man. I must admit that I was surprised to see someone who had been so effective in life so utterly demolished by something called depression. It took many months to restore him to health. During those months, his business suffered greatly. The impact of depression on job productivity is highlighted in the chapter by Jim Mintz and colleagues, in which they point out that the cost of depression to the United States economy is estimated to be more than $40 billion annually! Moreover, it causes a downward spiral; depression impairs work and the diminished ability to work induces more depression. The need to recognize and deal with depression in the workplace could not be more urgent. This need is central to rehabilitation, which involves the restoration of functional and work capacity and career guidance. Depression, if not recognized and successfully managed, can seriously impede such efforts, as Mary Ellen Copeland so aptly describes.

In the elderly, failure to diagnose depression may not only seriously interfere with a client's quality of life, but also increase his or her risk of physical illness — or even death. This is not surprising, when one considers the chapter by Elinor M.

Levy, Cheryl Chancellor-Freeland, and Richard Krueger, which describes the impact of depression on the human immune system. The value of two different approaches to counseling the elderly to minimize the impact of stress and depression are explored by Duane A. Lundervold and by Wanda Y. Johnson, respectively.

A special mental health problem is most likely to occur in elderly patients; namely, the existence of depression in patients who have suffered strokes. As Rajesh M. Parikh and Robert G. Robinson explain, depression is an aspect of the stroke patient's medical condition that is often overlooked, in spite of the fact that studies indicate a 30%-50% incidence rate of depression following a stroke. It's all too easy to ask oneself: "Who wouldn't be depressed if he or she had a stroke?" This question is natural enough. Unfortunately, however, this attitude can be seriously counterproductive; the fact is that patients who experience post-stroke depression recover more quickly and more fully when their depression is accurately diagnosed and appropriately treated—usually with antidepressant medications.

In clients of all ages, there is a high risk of misdiagnosing a serious physical illness as only a form of depression. The statistics are startling. Thirty-two percent of nonpsychiatric physicians, who should "know better" miss the diagnosis of an underlying medical illness when faced with depressive symptoms; 48% of psychiatrists and an astonishing 83% of nonmedical social agencies do the same. Mark S. Gold offers important warnings for any mental health professional working with depressed clients: Be sure your client has had a complete medical examination in the recent past. Be familiar with any conditions the client may have and any medications he or she may be taking. Finally, be on the alert for the emergence of health problems during the course of your therapy with all clients and patients.

We'll all be better able to keep special issues such as these in mind if we base our clinical approach to managing depression on a biopsychosocial model. We'll be in a stronger position to appreciate the important interrelationship between our psychological approaches to treatment and the appropriate use of antidepressant medications.

In the closing chapter of this useful guide, Pedro L. Delgado and Alan J. Gelenberg present an excellent discussion about when to choose to administer an antidepressant medication. They echo my own thinking about how antidepressants really work; namely that antidepressant agents do not seem to act specifically against major depression. My concept of psychobiological resilience (Flach, 1988, 1977/1995a, 1974/1995b) posits that, in most instances, depression itself is not the heart of the problem; the real problem lies in whether the mood is recognized and handled by depressed clients or patients and how successfully they can recover from a state of emotional disruption on their own. When improvement is unlikely without medication, when possible harmful effects (such as loss of employment, marital discord, or even suicide) may otherwise arise, or when the client has a strong family history of depression, antidepressants should be started early on. On the other hand, if symptoms are mild and responsive to psychotherapy, if the risk of harmful consequences is minimal, or if depression appears to be secondary to recent severe life stresses, medical illness, or coadministered medications, the use of antidepressants usually can be comfortably postponed or omitted altogether.

Because most people suffering from depression can and will recover, if the depression is properly managed—and having recovered, can become more insightful, stronger, and better able to cope for what they have been through—treating such clients can be an extremely gratifying and rewarding experience for most clinicians.

Frederic Flach, MD
New York

Dr. Flach is Adjunct Associate Professor of Psychiatry, Cornell University Medical College, New York; and Attending Psychiatrist at Payne Whitney Clinic of The New York Hospital and St. Vincent's Hospital and Medical Center, New York.

REFERENCES

Flach, F. (1988). *Resilience.* New York: Fawcett Columbine.

Flach, F. (1995a). *Putting the pieces together again: A physician's guide to thriving on stress.* New York: Hatherleigh Press. (Original work published 1977)

Flach, F. (1995b). *The secret strength of depression* (2nd rev. ed.). New York: Hatherleigh Press. (Original work published 1974)

1

Adaptive Styles in the Etiology of Depression

Peter C. Whybrow, MD

Dr. Whybrow is Professor and Chairman of the Department of Psychiatry at the University of Pennsylvania, Philadelphia, PA.

KEY POINTS

- The psychological management of the depressed client requires a careful understanding of the maladaptive behavior patterns that have set the stage for illness and may retard recovery.

- The close relationship between the quality of human attachments and vulnerability to depression/loss of self-esteem merits careful attention in the following areas: the development of autonomy, the role of attachment and separation, self-esteem and competence, and grief.

- Some persons never resolve the psychobiological issues surrounding attachment and separation and will thus develop a particular adaptive style to deal with disturbed attachment-separation issues and to protect against the impact of depression. Such adaptive styles include: dependence on a dominant person, excessive control, and pseudoindependence.

- It is essential for the clinician to detect the emergence of adaptive styles early so that an appropriate relationship with the client may be built and an effective method of treatment designed.

- Once the immediate, disorganizing elements in depression have been relieved, clients have an excellent opportunity to revise the adaptive mechanisms formed earlier in life and learn new and better modes of adaptation.

INTRODUCTION

Psychological mechanisms play a significant role in both the genesis and resolution of depression. Although psychodynamic factors may appear more apparent in so-called reactive depressions — those in which events of a specific and identifiable nature appear related to the onset of the episode of dysphoric mood — they cannot be ignored even in the treatment of clients whose symptoms are primarily of the melancholic type and in whom clear-cut precipitating causes may not be obvious. Whether the goals of treatment are limited and supportive or intensive and aimed at fundamental characterological changes, the psychological management of the depressed client requires a careful understanding of maladaptive behavior patterns that have set the stage for illness and may retard recovery.

It is generally accepted that a significant loss, frequently highly personalized, is commonly a cause for depression, particularly when such trauma involves a diminution of self-esteem. However, the manner in which a particular client has tended to cope with various losses over the years — the mode of adaptation — can take a number of different forms, each of which calls for an appropriate therapeutic strategy. To understand these styles, it seems logical to briefly review the close relationship between the quality of human attachments on the one hand and the vulnerability to depression and loss of self-esteem on the other.

NORMAL ADAPTATION AND THE DEVELOPMENT OF AUTONOMY

All living creatures maintain a relative autonomy from their environment. This is implemented by adaptation. In this regard, human beings do not differ from other organisms, except that they are more complex.

Adaptation is essentially the appropriate response of the

organism to an environmental challenge, whether it is an invading microorganism or a perceived psychic assault. When a person can adapt with some degree of success, this phenomenon is called "coping." From the perspective of practical psychobiology, we may view human depression as a temporary failure to adapt successfully—a state in which the person is transiently overwhelmed by diverse challenge. This is not necessarily pathological. In fact, it is the disruption and learned adaptations to various challenges early in life that make later coping possible. Exposure to infectious agents builds immunity. The complex dendritic structure of the cerebellum grows more complex under the challenge of learning how to walk. Innate ability is no less important than the quality of environmental events in this process of growth. However, the acquisition of coping ability is facilitated by consistency in the environmental challenge. Thus, an environment that is capricious, punitive, unpredictable, overprotective, or inadequate in its challenge usually will result in restricted styles of personality coping.

For the growing child, as for the adult, change is an everyday occurrence. One of the central issues in childhood involves the experience of separation and loss. As the child learns how to successfully master these issues, autonomy and an objective regard of self also are built. Feelings of helplessness and even hopelessness are integral parts of this development. Schmale and Engel (1975) called these "signal functions"—warnings to permit the anticipation of special traumas that have been experienced previously and now threaten to overwhelm the person unless successful adaptation is achieved.

THE ROLE OF ATTACHMENT AND SEPARATION

The significance of attachments in the formation of self-esteem and autonomy is not unique to human beings. In primates, for example, the reaction to separation is clearly defined. Close attachment between parent and offspring and, later, between peers is the developmental mode in primates. Once such attachment is formed, disruption causes a stage of protest and, subsequently, withdrawal, involving both a psychological detachment and a somatic withdrawal.

A similar syndrome, the response to separation from the caring parent, has been the object of considerable study in human infants. Attention was first specifically drawn to this phenomenon by Spitz and Wolf (1946), who focused largely on the withdrawal phase and termed it *anaclitic depression*. Later, Bowlby's studies (1973) and those of others made it apparent that the reaction to separation follows a typical pattern, best understood in sequence and essentially as follows:

During the first year of life, the child begins to form a specific attachment to the person who provides most of his or her care, as well as to the environment in which that care takes place. Most important, through the central nervous system, an awareness develops of the special association between subjective comfort and the events that occur. Thus, in a strange environment— and particularly in the presence of a stranger — the infant protests initially and then becomes tense and cries out. If the preferred person does not return, the protest continues; after awhile, however, it merges into what appears to be a despairing detachment. Schmale and Engel (1975) called this *conservation-withdrawal*, citing the example of an infant who had been fed through a gastric fistula with minimal nurturing because of her mother's depression. When her protest was exhausted, a phase of conservation-withdrawal became dominant—a passive, sleep-like state associated with virtually no motor activity and cessation of gastric secretion.

Such withdrawal appears to be an adaptive response to a depriving environment. It is an experience that is, to some degree, unavoidable in the life of any infant or child. In fact, if not too severe, traumatic, or prolonged, it is invaluable as a developmental challenge. As the child grows, the biological state becomes associated with subjective feelings of helplessness, to which feelings of hopelessness may be later added as the person consciously recognizes the inadequacy of his or her capacity to respond. This basic psychosomatic process stands in sharp contrast to the active-engaging posture that the growing infant adopts when secure in an environment perceived as nurturing.

In humans, the basic psychobiological process of attachment and separation is significantly modified by abstract conceptual thought. Our ability to adapt to and modify our environment in our own interest is a function of our particularly complex and vigilant nervous system that integrates and modulates every detail of our response. As we grow, we learn to tolerate separation and to supplement with others the exclusive caring originally provided by parents. Eventually, we provide our own needed supports and set standards that are both internal and specific to ourselves.

SELF-ESTEEM AND COMPETENCE

Self-esteem is a healthy respect for one's abilities and appreciation of one's limitations. Its regulation is perhaps one of the most complicated mechanisms in human psychology. There is no single road to a sense of mastery. Throughout life, we strive for autonomy and discover, in the process, ingenious ways to cope. Based on past experiences, we form ideals against which to measure achievement; self-esteem becomes, in large part, a function of the extent to which persons believe they can and do live up to the goals they have set for themselves. From a developmental point of view, it is critical to remember that the substructure that supports self-esteem, ego ideals, and autonomy in adult life derives from the nature of the bonds that were developed and subsequently modified during the person's childhood in relationships with members of his or her primary family.

As Bowlby (1973) pointed out:

> When an individual is confident that an attachment figure will be available to him when he deserves it, that person will be much less prone to either intense or chronic fear than will be an individual who for any reason has no such confidence.

Confidence in the accessibility and responsiveness to attachment figures, or lack of it, is built up slowly during all the years
of immaturity; and once developed, these expectations tend to
persist relatively unchanged throughout life.

Self-reliance is not, therefore, the cultural stereotype of
needing no one; rather, it is the ability to rely trustingly on
others, to know on whom to rely and when, and to permit
oneself to be relied upon.

GRIEF

Over a period of years, one's sense of self and of reality evolves
as one builds an analogue of the perceived world and then
embellishes it. This becomes a private template for adaptation
and the maintenance of autonomy, serving to help us cope
with the changes and losses that life inevitably provides, such
as leaving home, illness, romantic and sexual attachment and
loss, marriage, divorce, children, and the death of those close
to us. When we falter at times in these adaptations, it is natural
to reexperience to some degree the helplessness and hopelessness that we experienced as children who were faced with
situations that seemed to be more than we could cope with at
the time. Such subjective feelings are reported as depression.
The healthy person recognizes them, understands them,
struggles with them, and eventually recovers by means of his
or her own adaptive modes.
	Many of these features are seen in the normal experience of
grief—the reaction that follows the death or loss of someone
with whom one has enjoyed a close emotional bond. The
stages in the process of grief resemble those seen in depression. The initial reaction is disbelief or protest. Somatic distress and a preoccupation with the image of the dead person go
hand in hand. Subsequently, we may experience a transient
loss of the usual patterns in which we conduct our lives, with
some withdrawal and guilty speculation on what contribution

we have made to the person's death or unhappiness during his or her lifetime. However, even though these disturbances seem indistinguishable from depressive illness at times, most people accept the experience in themselves or in their friends and relatives as quite normal, providing they recover from the impact in a reasonable period and do not enter a serious psychiatric disorder.

MALADAPTIVE PERSONALITY STYLES AND DEPRESSION

Vulnerability to depressive illness seems to be increased in persons who, for whatever reason, have never satisfactorily resolved the psychobiological issues surrounding attachment and separation. Such persons remain extremely sensitive to loss — or perceived loss — whether of people, animals, their own career goals, philosophical aspirations, friendships, or material things.

Frequently, in defending against this contingency and its associated feelings of helplessness and hopelessness, such persons have acquired adaptive styles that are meant to aid them in coping but are, in fact, often setting them up to exchange a more normal period of grief for a serious episode of illness. The common denominator among these styles is rigidity. Some of the mechanisms — or rescue operations — may work quite well for years, but, at some point, often in middle age, a special combination of events may disrupt the precarious equilibrium and, with it, the person's self-esteem.

I have found it useful to cluster such adaptive types into three major, although somewhat overlapping, categories: dependence on a dominant person, excessive control, and pseudoindependence.

Dependence on a Dominant Person:

In this adaptive style, the basic rescue strategy is to transfer the unresolved issues surrounding attachment and separation from the parenting figures to others in the person's life who appear competent and capable. Thus, no true self-reliance develops during the maturing years, and the person enters adult life with a constricted series of adaptive options.

Persons who use this strategy find it difficult to enter the usual commerce of adult life, because their own self-esteem is tied too closely to the opinions of those around them. This does not mean that adaptation is impossible; in fact, sometimes it is quite successful for a long time. The key to their adequate psychosocial function, however, is dependence on some dominant figure who maintains a caretaker's role.

Traditionally, this form of working adaptation has been seen more commonly among women in our culture, possibly in part because it has been considered acceptable, perhaps even desirable, for women to be dependent on a dominant male figure. Often, such women married early, moved away from their primary families, and spent considerable energy trying to please the men on whom they depended for their self-worth. If their husbands reciprocated with kindness and support, this kind of balance could continue for years and was usually threatened when their role as mothers diminished as their children grew up and left home. More recently, however, it has been recognized that men can just as readily form such dependent attachments on women, leaving their primary homes without adequate autonomy and looking to their lovers or wives for parental support.

Such an adaptation can function, more or less, until the dominant figure in the person's life disrupts the primary bond, either by cruelty, desertion, infidelity, death, or some other intercurrent event. Unfortunately, persons who adapt in this way frequently form a liaison with persons who are struggling to ward off the pain of attachment-separation problems by means of pseudoindependence, a style described later on, and who have a need for support, but, by one means or another, have been able to rely on their own abilities exclusively early in their adult lives. Frequently, in such a marriage, as the man becomes increasingly engaged in a professional role, he is no longer able or willing to nurture his dependent wife; as a woman devotes more of her time to children or her own pursuits, her dependent husband feels abandoned.

Under these circumstances, the adaptive style starts to crack. The dedication and investment in the affairs of the family or the other bring diminishing rewards. As one partner or the other becomes increasingly remote, the vulnerable person feels a sense of growing helplessness and hopelessness that is identified as depression and that may well progress to severe illness. Anger, which has been present for a long time, erupts. The suppressed anger was basically driven by the vulnerable person's sense of never having been truly provided for or cared about, either in the primary family or within the present relationship. Withdrawal and serious depression may ensue.

Excessive Control:

When an inconsistency exists in the available caring figures during the maturational years, a potential adaptation in adolescence and early adult life is to reduce to a minimum the number of situations in which the difficult task of resolving separation anxiety is likely to occur. The need to control the day-to-day details of life becomes a primary mechanism of adaptation. Basic to this strategy is the restriction of novelty and the unexpected. Planning assumes great importance. Surprises are often greeted with a hostile response. In such a character structure, there is little spontaneity; instead, meticulousness and reliability are developed to an extreme. Because these obsessive styles are highly marketable and well rewarded, such people do fairly well early in life.

This adaptation is usually seen as a psychological rescue attempt in a person who has had little opportunity to develop a fundamental trust in others. It serves to compensate for an inadequate resolution of the attachment-separation paradigm. When the adaptive style is threatened by an increased number of events that the person can no longer keep under control, the underlying lack of trust rapidly appears. Overt suspiciousness and even paranoia may emerge, covering up the intense sense of helplessness that such persons usually feel. This, in turn, only isolates them even further from human contact.

Even when the strategy of control is working, such persons find it difficult to delegate authority to others. It is not uncommon for the very work habits that permit them to rise through organization ranks or in professions to become serious handicaps when positions of real authority and leadership are reached. They gradually fail as they become unable to control the steadily increasing number of variables with which they have to deal. Aging, illness, and other life problems that reduce the ability to remain in control shake the foundation of this defense against the pain of loss, leading to depression.

Pseudoindependence:

The pseudoindependence method of adaptation is closely allied with that of maintaining excessive control. Again, the person avoids close contact with others and thereby reduces the opportunities for loss. To all outward appearance, such persons appear independent, competent, with high aspirations for themselves and others. They may believe in a well-structured philosophy based on social or religious beliefs. They may enjoy serving others and usually do it well; hence, they are often valuable members of their communities. However, they often have broken away from their primary family early in life, setting up, by effort and hard work, an independent life of their own. Instinctively, they make others dependent on them, thereby gaining vicarious gratification and clearly feeling safer under such circumstances.

On the other hand, not far beneath the surface and usually within their awareness, they often yearn for a close relationship with a caring person—someone who fits the very ego ideal for which they themselves strive. Not infrequently, such persons marry someone similar to themselves and create a life together characterized by remoteness on an emotional level. Here again, illness, aging, and the departure of those who have been dependent on them — such as children growing up and leaving — represent special threats to their ability to cope. Because they are fearful of being dependent, they often resist seeking help until they have no choice left, and consulting a professional can represent an occasion of intense fear, even panic. In therapy, they are frequently resistant to complying with antidepressant medication if recommended, feeling further compromised in their effort to maintain independence.

ADAPTIVE STYLES AND THERAPY

The particular styles that clients have assumed during their lives to deal with disturbed attachment-separation issues and protect against the impact of depression will reflect themselves in the relationships that are formed with the clinicians and in the attitude the clients have in approaching treatment. Professionals must carefully note the emergence of such factors as early as possible in their contact with clients. Sometimes, as in the case of a client who has sought the protection of depending on a dominant other, finding an understanding and empathetic professional serves to restore a sense of security and worth, catalyzing recovery. There is, in some instances, a risk that clients will become too dependent on clinicians and unable to maintain improvement when the end of the therapeutic relationship is in sight. Clinicians must give clients the support that they need early on but simultaneously work to cultivate a greater degree of self-reliance as therapy progresses.

Distrustful, severely controlled clients can be particularly problematic. These clients often are reluctant to open up and communicate spontaneously with clinicians for fear of losing further control. Compliance with medication regimens is commonly difficult to obtain. In the course of sessions, clinicians' patience may be tried by perceived power struggles between themselves and their clients. These struggles actually represent clients' attempts to regain control over every aspect of their lives. Treating clients' symptoms with antidepressants often permits them to function more efficiently again and thus alleviates their distress and heightened need for control that derive from their strong sense of helplessness. However, because the goals that such clients set for themselves usually are unattainable, one of the major tasks in treatment is to help them accept the impossibility of their obsessive style and learn how to feel comfortable with uncertainty, ambiguity, and risk and how to gradually place greater trust in others who are worthy of it.

For clients whose style has been one of pseudoindependence, one of the main challenges in treatment is to help them accept whatever limitations life has forced on them and to learn how to permit themselves to rely on others.

Issues around attachment and separation, loss and its resolution, are obviously not the only way in which depression emerges. Many other factors, both social and biological, conspire with intrapsychic mechanisms to precipitate the final common path of dysfunction. Such dysfunction itself, however, can represent for depressed clients a unique pathway to growth and a singular opportunity to learn new and better adaptive styles.

Once the immediate, disorganizing elements in depression have been relieved, clients have an excellent opportunity to work with clinicians to rethink some of the rescue mechanisms that they developed automatically in earlier years. Although many of these mechanisms may have served them well, others clearly have done them disservice. This is the time to acquire additional rescue mechanisms, in particular mechanisms that will provide the flexibility needed by depressed clients to cope more effectively with challenges in their present and future lives.

REFERENCES

Bowlby, J. (1973). *Attachment and loss II: Separation.* New York: Basic Books.

Schmale, A., & Engel, G. (1975). The role of conservation-withdrawal in depressive reactions. In A. Jones & T. Benedek (Eds.). *Depression and human existence.* Boston, MA: Little Brown & Company.

Spitz, R., & Wolf, K. (1946). Anaclitic depression. In *Psychoanalytic study of the child* (Vol. 2, pp. 313-342). New York: International Universities Press.

FOR FURTHER READING

Coopersmith, S. (1967). *The antecedents of self-esteem.* San Francisco: Freeman.

Epstein, S. (1976). Anxiety, arousal and self concept. In T. G. Saranon & C. D. Spolberger (Eds.), *Stress and anxiety* (Vol. III). Washington, DC: Hemisphere.

Whybrow, P. C., Aksikal, H., & McKinney, W. J. (1984). *Mood disorders: Toward a new psychobiology.* New York: Plenum Press.

2

Depression and the Immune System

Elinor M. Levy, PhD, Cheryl Chancellor-Freeland, PhD, and
Richard Krueger, MD

Dr. Levy is Associate Professor of Microbiology and Dr. Chancellor-Freeland is Immunology Fellow in the Department of Microbiology at Boston University School of Medicine, Boston, MA. Dr.
Krueger is Assistant Clinical Professor of Psychiatry at Columbia
College of Physicians and Surgeons, New York, NY, and an
attending psychiatrist at Columbia Presbyterian Hospital and the
New York State Psychiatric Institute, New York, NY.

KEY POINTS

- The immune system and the brain can interact. This interaction may influence disease processes.

- The central players of the immune system are the lymphocytes, which provide specificity and memory through the various B cells, T cells, and null cells, each of which plays a different functional role.

- Some studies on the immune status of depressed patients suggest that greater depression is associated with more suppressed immune function, whereas other studies indicate the elevation of some immune functions in depression.

- Although depression offers the opportunity to study the relationship between psychological status and the immune response, some caution must be taken when evaluating such a relationship. Behavioral changes caused by depression, such as smoking, sleep deprivation, dietary changes, and medications, may also affect the immune response.

- Continued study of the association between depression and immune suppression should elucidate one pathway for the transformation of psychological factors into increased morbidity.

INTERACTIONS BETWEEN THE BRAIN AND THE IMMUNE SYSTEM

There is a popular belief that the mind can determine suscep- tibility to disease. Evidence from clinical studies and animal models supporting this concept has been reviewed (Dantzer & Kelly, 1989; Gorman & Locke, 1989). The data indicating a role for the psyche in influencing both the severity and incidence of infectious disease, particularly viral infections, are convinc- ing. Intriguing data suggesting associations between the mind and autoimmune diseases, including allergies and cancer, are also available. In most of these studies, psychological factors, such as stress or an inability to cope with stress, have been linked to an increase in the incidence or severity of illness. Other studies, however, indicate that stress can be protective under certain circumstances.

In recent years, attention has focused on changes in the immune system as a mechanism by which psychological fac- tors can influence disease processes. The immune system seems a reasonable choice for transforming psychological signals into somatic ones. First, in all the aforementioned diseases, the immune system plays a potentially prominent role. Ample evidence also exists demonstrating that the im- mune system is sensitive to neuroendocrine hormones and transmitters. Thus, disregulated immune function can be ex- pected to alter susceptibility to these diseases. Immune reac- tivity is modified by glucocorticosteroids, adrenocorticotropic hormone (ACTH), the endorphins and enkephalins, catechola- mines, and acetylcholine. This is a fact largely ignored by immunologists. Marx (1985) pointed out that it is time for immunologists to recognize that the immune system "belongs in the body."

A fascinating body of evidence shows that the immune system can influence the mind. For example, following an antigenic challenge, the neuronal firing rate in the hypothala- mus increases, as do plasma cortisol levels (Besedovsky et al., 1983). This increase in cortisol may be in response to an ACTH-like molecule that activated lymphocytes can produce (Smith & Blalock, 1981). Thus, it seems clear that the immune system and the brain can interact, and that this interaction might well influence disease processes.

Although this concept has great theoretical appeal, it has been difficult to document in human beings. Animal models, however, have clearly demonstrated that psychological stress can increase the growth of tumors and susceptibility to infections. Such models also show that the same stressors reduce immune function. Although many parallels exist between human and murine immune systems, some important differences are also evident. One such example is the different ways the two systems respond to glucocorticosteroids. Thus, one must be cautious when extrapolating from research performed in mice to humans.

In humans, work in this area is hampered by natural variability among persons, the enormous complexity of the immune system, and the formidable complexity of the neuroendocrine system. A promising new approach to this problem has been to focus on clients with major psychiatric depression. The severity and duration of this condition allow significant differences in immune function to be correlated with alterations in neuroendocrine hormone levels. Results of research in this area are reviewed later in this chapter.

THE IMMUNE SYSTEM: AN OVERVIEW

The immune system acts to protect us from a large variety of pathogens and toxins. It first recognizes these elements as foreign and then uses one of several mechanisms at its disposal to eliminate or inactivate them. Immune responses are divided into those that involve antibody (termed *humoral responses*) and those that involve cell-mediated immunity. In addition to pathogens, the immune system has the capability to recognize and destroy transformed or cancerous cells. It can, with some cancers, also protect against the growth and metastasis of tumor cells. However, the immune system is not infallible, as those of us with allergies or autoimmune disease can attest. The list of diseases classified as autoimmune continues to grow and includes rheumatoid arthritis, myasthenia gravis, and certain forms of diabetes and asthma. To prevent misplaced reactivity and to limit the exuberance of otherwise appropriate immune reactions, the immune system includes a variety of checks and balances. A brief overview of the components of the immune system and how they interact is given below.

The immune system is remarkably complex. Its central players are the lymphocytes, which provide specificity and memory. Each lymphocyte can respond to only one or a closely related set of antigenic determinants. Having been stimulated by its appropriate antigen, some lymphocytes differentiate to become memory cells. Memory cells are more sensitive than naïve lymphocytes and respond rapidly to subsequent encounters with antigen. Other lymphocytes differentiate into effector or regulatory cells after an encounter with antigen.

The lymphocytes are divided into *B cells*, *T cells*, and *null cells* (see Table 2.1). B cells produce antibodies, T cells provide specific cell-mediated immunity, and null cells can provide a quick but nonspecific form of cell-mediated immunity. B cells are, in turn, subdivided according to the type of immunoglobulin they carry on their surface (i.e., IgM, IgD, IgG, IgA, or IgE). The different antibody classes have different functional roles. IgA, for instance, is released into secretory fluids and may be particularly important in preventing respiratory infections. Antibodies, in general, coat pathogens and help inactivate or target them for destruction by the granulocytes and the reticuloendothelial system.

T cells are subdivided into functional subgroups: helper, inducer, suppressor, and cytotoxic T cells. To a large extent, T cells can be classified by the surface antigens they possess. Helper and inducer cells are generally positive for the CD4 antigen; suppressor and cytotoxic cells are generally positive for the CD8 antigen.

Table 2.1
CELLS OF THE IMMUNE SYSTEM

Cells	Cell Markers	Cell Products	Function
Lymphocytes B Cells	IgM, IgD, IgG, IgE, IgA	Antibodies	Antibodies inactivate some viruses and bacteria and target other pathogens for destruction by other cells of the immune system
T Cells	CD3, CD2, CD4, or (on helper/inducer cells) CD8 (on cytoxic/suppressor cells)	Lymphokines (e.g., IL-2, interferon, TNF (tumor necrosis factor)	Regulate function of B cells, effector T cells, and macrophage; cytoxic T cells kill infected host cells and neoplastic cells
NK Cells	HNK-1	Interferon, perforin	Kill certain virally infected and neoplastic cells
Macrophages	CD14, la	IL-1, interferon, H_2O_2, prostaglandins	Bactericidal, tumoricidal, accessory role in immune reactions

Null cells are a heterogeneous collection of lymphoid cells that cannot be classified as B or T cells. They include immature T and B cells as well as natural killer cells. *Natural killer (NK) cells* can kill certain tumor and virally infected cells. In animal models, NK cells can be shown to be important in the early stages of certain viral infections and in clearing certain tumor cells, particularly from the lungs.

The T cells orchestrate the immune response. Let us consider antibody production as an example. Although B cells can recognize antigens directly, they require additional signals, provided by T helper cells, to proliferate and differentiate into memory or antibody-secreting plasma cells. The T helper cells not only stimulate B cells, but also amplify the antibody response by inducing proliferation and differentiation of other relevant T helper cells. T inducer cells help control the reaction by activating suppressor cells that can then turn off T helper cell activity. T cells produce factors such as immune (gamma) interferon and interleukin-2 (IL-2 or T cell growth factor), called lymphokines or cytokines. The cytokines are now recognized as important immunoregulatory molecules that allow immune cells to communicate with each other as well as with nonimmune cells, including those in neuroendocrine tissues.

In some situations, other T cells can be activated to become cytotoxic cells. These cells can kill pathogens, host cells infected with viruses or other intracellular pathogens, and transformed cells. T cells can also activate other cells, such as macrophages, to become bactericidal or tumoricidal.

Monocytes and macrophages are important in the initial stages of an immune response when they act as accessory cells. These cells process antigen, present in a particularly antigenic form to T cells, and produce factors that stimulate B and T cells. At other times, macrophages that have become activated can act as suppressor cells and inhibit the immune response through the release of suppressive factors, such as prostaglandin E. Other cells, including B cells and activated endothelial cells, can also serve as antigen presenting cells.

Thus, the immune system includes both effector and regulatory cells that interact to produce humoral and/or cell-mediated responses. Contact with antigen will stimulate a network of reactions. The end result depends on which of these pathways predominate. This in turn depends on the number and type of competent cells available for interaction.

MEASUREMENTS OF IMMUNOCOMPETENCE

A variety of tests are used to try to assess general immunocompetence. One such measure is performed in vivo. It measures the delayed type hypersensitivity reaction to five to seven commonly encountered antigens. It requires antigen recognition, migration, and activation of T helper cells and macrophages.

A simpler measure of immunocompetence is the in-vivo mitogen test. *Mitogens* are substances, such as the plant-derived phytohemagglutinin (PHA) or concanavalin A (conA), which stimulate lymphocytes to divide. PHA and conA are called *T-cell mitogens* because they stimulate the majority of T cells. Mitogenesis requires T-cell–macrophage cooperation and the production of many of the same factors needed to produce effective humoral or cell-mediated immunity. One usually quantitates activation by the amount of radioactive thymidine that cells incorporate when cultured in the presence of mitogen. Other mitogens, such as pokeweed mitogen (PWM), predominantly stimulate B cells to proliferate but require T cells as helpers. An alternative test that more closely mimics antigen stimulation involves activating T lymphocytes with an antibody (anti CD3), the latter acting as part of the antigen receptor activation complex. Again, proliferation is measured as a sign of responsiveness.

The quantitation of lymphokine production in response to a stimulus is another measure of immunocompetence. Cytokines can be assessed using bioassays, which rely on a quantifiable response to the cytokine. Alternatively, kits exist for measuring most cytokines using an ELISA (enzyme-linked immunosorbent assay) kit. Measuring cytokine specific mRNA is also used to assess cytokine production.

NK-cell activity is measured as the release of an isotope, such as chromium, from labeled sensitive target cells. Most commonly, the tumor-cell line, arbitrarily called K562, is used as a target cell. The damaged cells release isotope into the culture supernatant, which is then counted in a gamma counter. The percentage of target cells killed is a measure of NK-cell activity.

An additional assessment of immune status can be obtained from the quantitation of the number or proportion of CD4 (helper/inducer) and CD8 (suppressor/cytotoxic) cells. Although moderate changes in the overall CD4/CD8 ratio may not mean that much, major changes tend to indicate a severely disregulated immune system. In acquired immunodeficiency syndrome (AIDS), for instance, a retrovirus infects CD4 cells and leads to a gradual reduction in their number. Some believe this is the major event in the pathogenesis of AIDS that leaves its victims unable to combat infections from opportunistic organisms. Other antigens, such as CD3 or CD2, can be used to measure the total number of T cells present.

INTERACTION OF THE IMMUNE SYSTEM WITH THE NEUROENDOCRINE SYSTEM

The immune system is responsive to regulation by a number of neuroendocrine hormones (see Table 2.2). The effects of the glucocorticosteroids have been studied extensively. In certain species, such as rats and mice, corticosteroids actually destroy immature T cells. This, however, is not the case in humans (Cupps & Fauci, 1982). In humans, glucocorticosteroids are generally immunosuppressive when given at high doses. Both lymphocyte migration patterns and lymphocyte and macrophage function are affected. The effect of the glucocorticosteroids depends on the subset examined, the location of the population studied, and the time of addition of steroid relative to antigen. In mice, for instance, the antibody response in the spleen is suppressed at the same time that the antibody response in the bone marrow is enhanced following steroid administration in vivo. This is, in part, probably due to the redistribution of competent cells. Glucocorticosteroids suppress secretion of early activation factors by lymphocytes and macrophages. However, in certain models, dexamethasone can, in fact, enhance antibody responses because of a differential effect on suppressor cell activity; that is, by inhibiting suppressor cells, the net reaction is augmented. Thus, at moderate doses, the effects of steroids can be rather complicated.

Other hypothalamic-pituitary-adrenal (HPA) mediators, such as ACTH and corticotropin-releasing hormone (CRH),

Table 2.2

THE INFLUENCE OF NEUROENDOCRINE HORMONES
AND TRANSMITTERS ON LYMPHOCYTE FUNCTION*

Suppressors	Enhancers
ACTH	Acetylcholine
CRH	Arginine vasopressin
Epinephrine	CRH
Endorphins	Endorphins
Glucocorticosteroids	Enkephalins
Norepinephrine	Glucocorticosteroids
Serotonin	Growth hormone
Somatostatin	Insulin
Vasoactive intestinal	Oxytocin
Peptide	Prolactin
	Substance P

*Note: Certain modulators, such as the endorphins and glucocorticosteroids, can either enhance or suppress immune function depending on their dose, time of addition, and type of function assayed.

can also influence immunity. CRH is especially interesting in that elevated CRH levels in the brain are associated with immunosuppression. The effect is thought to be secondary to the effect of CRH on other neuroendocrine compounds, such as the catecholamines. Elevated CRH in the periphery is associated with immune stimulation and inflammation. Elevated levels of CRH are detected in inflamed joints.

Catecholamines can also influence both the function and distribution of lymphocytes. Catecholamines have been reported to suppress antibody production when added to lymphocyte cultures but to enhance NK-cell activity if cells are preincubated with norepinephrine. In vivo, their effect seems to be caused in part by their ability to change the distribution of lymphocytes. Crary and colleagues (1983) reported that the injection of epinephrine into volunteers caused a rapid increase in the total number of lymphocytes in the peripheral blood. There was a relative decrease in the proportion of CD4 cells, and a relative increase in the proportion of NK cells. Cells drawn at this time for in-vitro testing had a reduced ability to proliferate in response to the T-cell mitogen PHA. However, adding epinephrine to mitogen cultures in vitro or preincubating cells with the catecholamine prior to mitogenic stimulation had no effect. This suggests that the in-vivo effect of epinephrine on the mitogen response was due to the change in the relative proportion of the lymphocyte subsets in the circulation, rather than to a direct effect of epinephrine on the lymphocytes. The alterations caused by a bolus of epinephrine in vivo were maximal at 30 minutes and had returned to normal by 2 hours. Alternatively, in-vivo administration of epinephrine could induce other neuroendocrine changes that could secondarily affect mitogenesis.

Neuropeptides also have been shown to have immuno-modulatory properties. Both the endorphins and enkephalins can influence immune function; however, the literature is somewhat contradictory. Beta-endorphin is reported to stimulate or suppress mitogenesis. Alpha-endorphin and the enkephalins reportedly suppress in-vitro antibody synthesis. NK-cell activity is also modulated by beta-endorphin. In-vitro beta-endorphin can stimulate NK-cell activity, but the effect is not mediated via an opiate receptor. In contrast, in-vivo experiments where electrical shocks were given in a particular protocol resulted in reduced NK-cell activity (Shavit & Martin, 1987). The effect could be blocked by naloxone (Narcan), suggesting that the effect was mediated by endogenous opiates binding to opiate receptors. (Both lymphocytes and macrophages have opiate receptors.) Additional work also suggests that endogenous opiates may influence immune status in vivo. Injection of leucine enkephalin or methionine enkephalin was shown to cause an increase in thymic and a decrease in splenic weight in mice (Plotnikoff, Murgo, & Faith, 1984).

ALTERATIONS IN THE LEVELS OF NEUROENDOCRINE HORMONES IN DEPRESSION

Alterations in the hypothalamic-pituitary-adrenal axis are the most extensively studied pieces of evidence for neuroendocrine abnormalities in depressed patients. It is known that some depressed patients have abnormally high levels of cortisol in their circulation. In some studies, as many as 70% of very depressed patients showed resistance to the suppressive effects of dexamethasone on cortisol production compared with, at most, 10% of normal control subjects (Rothschild, 1988). It has been suggested that this may be a result of decreased concentrations of serotonin and catecholamines in the hypothalamus in depressed patients.

Other abnormalities in the hypothalamic-pituitary-adrenal axis have been reported in depressed patients. Patients had a reduced ACTH output in response to infused corticotropin-releasing factor (CRF) but, nonetheless, responded with a slightly greater than normal amount of cortisol secretion (Holsboer et al., 1984). In another study, by Nemeroff and colleagues (1984), the level of CRF-like material in cerebral spinal fluid was elevated in a group of patients with major depression but not in patients with schizophrenia or senile dementia.

IMMUNE STATUS IN DEPRESSED PATIENTS

A number of studies of immune status in depressed patients have been conducted (see Table 2.3). In one of their early studies, Kronfol and associates (1983) evaluated 26 patients hospitalized for depression who were drug free for at least 2 weeks prior to the study. Their mean score was 16.3 on the 17-item Hamilton Depression Rating Scale. The group had a reduced proliferative response to both the T-cell mitogens, conA and PHA, as well as to the T-dependent B-cell mitogen PWM. There was a nonsignificant trend for more-depressed patients to have lower mitogen responses than less-depressed patients. The authors stated that there was no difference in the responses of patients who had been taking medications prior to the 2-week drug-free period preceding the study and those

---

Table 2.3

IMMUNE CHANGES IN DEPRESSED PATIENTS

Study	Changes
T. Kronfol et al. (1983)	Decreased mitogenesis
S. Schleifer et al. (1984)	Decreased mitogenesis, decrease in T- and B-cell numbers
M. Stein et al. (1991)	Variable changes in mitogenesis and NK-cell activity
E. Levy et al. (1991)	Decreased mitogenesis, but only in major depression
M. Irwin et al. (1990)	Decreased NK-cell activity
M. Maes et al. (1993)	Increased IL-1 levels in depression

---

who had not; that is, if there was an effect due to medications, 2 weeks without drugs appeared to be sufficient to eliminate that effect.

Schleifer and colleagues (1984), in a later study of 18 hospitalized depressed patients, also noted a reduced response to the mitogens conA, PHA, and PWM, as compared with age- and sex-matched controls. These patients had not used drugs for at least 2 weeks prior to the study. Their mean Hamilton Depression Score was 28. The study also noted a decrease in the absolute numbers of peripheral blood B and T cells, although there did not appear to be a change in the relative proportion of B and T cells. In this study, rosetting techniques were used to enumerate B and T cells. Cortisol levels were significantly elevated in the depressed patients (14.05 μg/dL compared with 8.62 μg/dL for controls). The authors noted that the observed changes appeared to be independent of the length of hospitalization prior to assessment of immune status, suggesting that the acute stress of hospitalization was not responsible for the results. Hospitalized patients generally tend to have elevated cortisol levels.

Krueger and colleagues (1984), in a study of 6 patients hospitalized for depression, examined changes in the lymphocyte subset distributions. The mean Hamilton Depression Score was 26.8. There was a significant decrease in the proportion of CD4 (helper/inducer) and CD2 (total T cells) cells, as judged by immunofluorescence with monoclonal antibodies. The proportion of B cells, CD8 cells (suppressor/cytotoxic), and NK cells was unchanged. These findings could help explain the decreased mitogen responses noted in the other studies, because a decreased proportion of CD4 cells would be expected to reduce the mitogen response.

Decreased mitogenesis and NK-cell activity are confirmed in some studies but not in others. A study by Levy and colleagues (1991) found that mitogen response to conA was lower for inpatients with major depression than it was for healthy controls or inpatients with other forms of depression. NK activity and CD4 and CD8 percentages did not differ among the patient groups or their controls. The Hamilton Depression Score was similar for the two patient groups. This would further support the view that depression is associated with lower immune function in only certain subsets of depressed patients.

These contradictions were discussed by Levy and Chancellor-Freeland (1995). A meta-analysis by Herbert and Cohen (1993) of papers on immunity and depression concluded that mitogen responsiveness and NK-cell activity are both reduced in depression with effect sizes ranging from 0.24-0.45. Evidence suggests that the greater the depression, the more suppressed the immune function. Hospitalized patients were more affected than nonhospitalized patients. There were also effects on a number of leukocyte numbers in the blood, including the number but not percentage of various lymphocyte subsets.

A series of intriguing studies by Maes and colleagues (e.g., 1993) indicate that some immune functions, notably those relating to macrophage inflammatory function, are elevated in depression. They further hypothesize that the hyperactivity of macrophages could contribute to the severity of depression by increasing HPA activation in a well-established feedback loop from the immune system to the central nervous system (Reichlin, 1993).

POSSIBLE CONFOUNDING FACTORS ASSOCIATED WITH DEPRESSION

Although depression offers an opportunity to study the relationship between psychological status and the immune response, several cautions should be noted. The immune response may be affected by a number of behavioral changes that may be associated with depression. These include heavy drinking, heavy smoking, sleeplessness, dietary changes, and medications.

Drinking can cause decreased NK-cell activity in alcoholics, but these changes are also associated with liver damage and nutritional deficiencies (Charpentier et al., 1984). Abnormalities in humoral immunity also have been reported. Acute high levels of blood alcohol would be expected to have a temporary inhibitory effect on immune function in vivo. In studies of the effect of alcohol on immune function in vitro, levels of 0.5%–2.0% alcohol depressed NK-cell and cytotoxic function. The effect depended on the continued presence of alcohol, in that cells that were preincubated with alcohol and then washed regained normal function. Irwin and associates (1990) showed alcoholism and depression are both associated with low NK-cell activity. Alcoholics and depressed patients each had low NK activity, and depressed patients with an alcohol dependency had still lower NK activity.

In several studies, smoking has been associated with decreased immune status. A habit of heavy smoking was associated with a modest decrease of CD4/CD8 ratios (Miller et al., 1982). This was caused by both a decrease in the proportion of CD4 cells and an increase in the proportion of CD8 cells. Neither the total number nor the proportion of T cells changed.

The CD4/CD8 ratio returned to normal in heavy smokers who gave up smoking for 6 weeks. The effects in moderate smokers were not significant. In another study, smoking more than 10 cigarettes a day was associated with decreased NK-cell activity and mitogen responses (Hersey, Prendergast, & Edwards, 1983). Again, smokers who were tested after they stopped smoking showed an improvement in immune function. The effects reported have been less pronounced than those observed in depression. Thus, it is possible that heavy smoking could contribute to the observed changes in depression. As far as we know, this has yet to be examined.

Sleep deprivation also can lead to decreased mitogen responsiveness. In studies by Palmblad and colleagues (1979), subjects were kept awake for 64 hours. Their mitogen response returned to normal within 5 days. More recently, Irwin (1992) showed that NK-cell activity decreased with insomnia or sleep disturbances, as assessed by sleep time, sleep efficiency, and non-REM (rapid eye movement) duration. The effect was seen both in controls and depressed patients.

Changes in dietary habits might also influence the immune response, but again effects are difficult to demonstrate except in extreme situations. It is known that protein-calorie malnutrition causes decreases in mitogenesis and decreases the CD4/CD8 ratio in children. These changes are accompanied by elevated serum cortisol levels. Deficiencies in single elements, such as zinc and vitamins A and E, can also depress immune function, as can high levels of dietary fats, particularly the polyunsaturated fatty acids.

Medications likely to be used to treat depression and their influence on the immune system are not well studied. Antidepressants that affect catecholamine turnover may very well have some effect on immune function. However, the studies of Kronfol and colleagues (1983) and Schleifer and colleagues (1984) in drug-free patients suggest that although the use of drugs should be taken into account, there are significant effects in depressed patients that are independent of medication.

CONCLUSION

Modern technology has afforded us a heretofore unavailable capacity to study the immune system. Radioimmune assays have also greatly enhanced the ability to measure neuroendocrine mediators. A new and exciting area of research is the exploration of the relationship between psychological, behavioral, and psychobiological factors with the immune system. One way of exploring the relationship is to assess immune function in depressed patients. Although such studies are few and must take into account the extraordinary number of factors that have been demonstrated to affect immune function, they suggest that depression is associated with immune suppression. Continued study of this association should elucidate one pathway for the transformation of psychological factors into increased morbidity.

REFERENCES

Besedovsky, H., et al. (1983). The immune response evokes changes in brain noradrenergic neurons. *Science, 221*, 564–565.

Charpentier, B., et al. (1984). Deficient natural killer cell activity in alcoholic cirrhosis. *Clinical and Experimental Immunology, 58*, 107–115.

Crary, B., et al. (1983). Epinephrine-induced changes in the distribution of lymphocyte subsets in peripheral blood of humans. *Journal of Immunology, 131*, 1178–1181.

Cupps, T., & Fauci, A. (1982). Corticosteroid-mediated immunoregulation in man. *Immunological Review, 65*, 133–150.

Dantzer, R., & Kelly, K. W. (1989). Stress and immunity: An integrated view of relationships between the brain and the immune system. *Life Sciences, 44*, 1995–2008.

Gorman, J. R., & Locke, S. E. (1989). Neural, endocrine, and immune interactions. In H. I. Kaplan, & B. J. Sadock (Eds.), *Comprehensive Textbook of Psychiatry/V* (Vol. 1., pp. 111–125). Baltimore: Williams & Wilkins.

Herbert, T. B., & Cohen, S. (1993). Depression and immunity: a meta-analytic review. *Psychological Bulletin, 113,* 471-486.

Hersey, P., Prendergast, D., & Edwards, A. (1983). Effects of cigarette smoking on the immune system. *Medical Journal of Australia, 2,* 425–429.

Holsboer, F., et al. (1984). Blunted corticotropin and normal cortisol response to human corticotropin-releasing factor in depression. *New England Journal of Medicine, 311,* 1127.

Irwin, M., et al. (1990). Major Depression Disorder, alcoholism, and reduced natural killer cell cytotoxicity. *Archives of General Psychology, 47,* 713-719.

Irwin, M., et al. (1992). Electroencephalographic sleep and natural killer activity in depressed patients and control subjects. *Psychosomatic Medicine, 54,* 10-21.

Kronfol, T., et al. (1983). Impaired lymphocyte function in depressive illness. *Life Sciences, 33,* 241–247.

Krueger, R., et al. (1984). Lymphocyte subsets in patients with major depression: Preliminary findings. *Advances, 1,* 5–9.

Levy, E. M., & Chancellor-Freeland, C. (1995). Immunomodulation associated with depression and stress. In R. Watson (Ed.), *Alcohol, Drugs of Abuse, & Immune Functions* (pp. 1-16). New York: CRC Press.

Levy, E. M., et al. (1991). Biological measures and cellular immunologic function in depressed psychiatric inpatients. *Psychological Research, 36,* 157–167.

Maes, M., et al. (1993). Interleukin-1ß: A putative mediator of HPA hyperactivity in major depression? *American Journal of Psychiatry, 150,* 1189-1193.

Marx, J. (1985). The immune system 'belongs in the body.' *Science, 227,* 1190-1192.

Miller, L., et al. (1982). Reversible alterations in immunoregulatory T cells in smoking. *Chest, 5,* 526–529.

Nemeroff, C., et al. (1984). Elevated concentrations of CRF corticotropin-releasing factor-like immunoreactivity in depressed patients. *Science, 226,* 1342–1344.

Palmblad, J., et al. (1979). Lymphocyte and granulocyte reactions during sleep deprivation. *Psychosomatic Medicine, 41,* 273–277.

Plotnikoff, N., Murgo, A., & Faith, R. (1984). Neuroimmunomodulation with enkephalins: Effects on thymus and spleen weights in mice. *Clinical Immunology and Immunopathology, 32,* 52-56.

Reichlin, S. (1993). Neuroendocrine-immune interactions. *New England Journal of Medicine, 329,* 1246-1251.

Rothschild, A. J. (1988). Biology of depression. *Medical Clinics of North America, 72,* 765-790.

Schleifer, S., et al. (1984). Lymphocyte function in major depressive disorder. *Archives of General Psychiatry, 41,* 484–486.

Shavit, Y., & Martin, F. (1987). Opiates, stress, and immunity: Animal studies. *Annals of Behavioral Medicine, 9,* 11-15.

Smith, E., & Blalock, J. (1981). Human lymphocyte production of corticotropin and endorphin-like substances: Association with leukocyte interferon. *Proceedings of the National Academy of Sciences of the United States of America, 78,* 7530–7534.

Stein, M., Miller, A., & Trestman, R. (1991). Depression, the immune system, and health and illness. *Archives of General Psychiatry, 48,* 171-177.

FOR FURTHER READING

Ader, R., Felten, D. L., & Cohen, N. (1991). *Psychoneuroimmunology* (2nd ed.). New York: Academic Press.

3

Post-Stroke Depression

Rajesh M. Parikh, MD, and Robert G. Robinson, MD

Dr. Parikh is Associate Professor, Jaslok Hospital and Research Center, Bombay, India. Dr. Robinson is Professor and Head, Department of Psychiatry, University of Iowa College of Medicine, Iowa City, IA.

KEY POINTS

- Post-stroke depression is unrecognized and untreated in most patients.

- Investigation of the emotional disorders associated with stroke may not only further our knowledge of the sequelae of stroke but may also advance our understanding of the brain mechanisms involved in regulating mood and behavior.

- A strong association exists between the frequency and severity of post-stroke depression and the location of brain injury. In comparison, a relatively weak relationship exists between physical and intellectual impairment and depression.

- Post-stroke depression can be treated through early and accurate diagnosis, careful use of medication, and counseling. It helps to improve the process of physical as well as emotional recovery.

- It is vital to understand all the mechanisms of the various post-stroke depressions in order to realize rational treatments. Moreover, the impact of the treatment of depression on the intellectual and physical recovery and social functioning of patients with stroke merits greater exploration.

INTRODUCTION

Stroke, defined as a sudden, nonconvulsive, focal neurologic deficit produced by an insufficiency of blood to the brain, is one of the major health problems in the United States (Adams & Victor, 1985). In addition to being the third leading cause of death and a major cause of physical disability among the elderly, stroke also has serious repercussions on the emotional and intellectual functioning of those who survive.

Although the physical signs and symptoms of stroke have been extensively documented and studied over the years, only recently has interest in the emotional consequences of stroke emerged. Yet, investigation of the emotional disorders associated with stroke may not only further our knowledge of the sequelae of stroke but may also advance our understanding of the brain mechanisms involved in regulating mood and behavior.

HISTORICAL BACKGROUND

The association between brain injury and mood disorders has been known for about a century. In 1904, Adolf Meyer described the "traumatic insanities" and postulated that they may have a relationship to specific areas of brain injury. Bleuler (1951) reported persistent, refractory depression following stroke, and Kraeplin (1921) discussed the etiological role of cerebrovascular disease in producing states of depression. More recently, Roth (1955) suggested injury to certain brain areas may produce depression.

Many clinicians, however, have assumed depression to be an understandable reaction to the impairments produced by stroke, rather than an integral feature of the disease itself. For example, Fisher (1961) stated the brain is the most cherished organ of the body and injury to it would understandably lead to depression. Systematic studies, however, tend to refute that assumption. For instance, Folstein and Maiberger (1977) found stroke patients were significantly more depressed than ortho-pedic patients with equal degrees of physical impairment. Finkelstein, Benowitz, and Baldessarini (1982) reported that symptoms of clinical depression as well as failure to suppress cortisol following dexamethasone administration were significantly more common in stroke patients when com-pared with a control group of patients with a variety of chronic medical illnesses. Our studies have also found only a weak correlation between depression and severity of either intel-lectual or physical impairment.

Prevalence:

Several studies have shown a 30%–50% incidence of post-stroke depression (Collin, Tinson, & Lincoln, 1987; Ebrahim, Baser, & Norin, 1987; Feibel & Springer, 1982; Haroon, 1986; Robinson et al., 1983; Robinson & Price, 1982; Sinyor et al., 1986; Wade, Legh-Smith, & Hewer, 1987). Of 103 outpatients who were seen at varying intervals post-stroke, we found 30% were depressed (Robinson & Price, 1982). Feibel and Springer (1982) reported a 26% incidence of depression in 91 outpa-tients seen 6 months after a stroke. Our study of 103 hospital-ized acute stroke patients revealed 47% were depressed, 27% with major depression and 20% with minor depression (Robinson et al., 1983). Sinyor and associates (1986) reported 49% of stroke patients admitted to a rehabilitation hospital had depressive symptoms. In India, Haroon (1986) found moderate-to-severe depressive mood in 20 of 40 stroke pa-tients. From the United Kingdom, Ebrahim and colleagues (1987) reported a 46% incidence of post-stroke depression, and Wade and co-workers (1987) found that 3 weeks after a stroke, 22% of outpatients were depressed and another 11% were probably depressed. In a community sample of 89 patients examined 1 month following stroke, House, Dennis, Mogridge, Warlow, and Jones (1991) found that 11% had major depression and 12% had minor depression (adjustment disorder). Finally, Collin and colleagues (1987) reported a prevalence of post-stroke depression in 42% of patients seen 1 and 2 years post-stroke.

Symptomatology:

The symptoms of post-stroke depression are phenomenologically similar to those seen in patients with depression of functional origin (i.e., with no known neuropathology) (Lipsey et al., 1986). Patients with post-stroke depression experience sadness, hopelessness, guilt, difficulties in thinking and concentration, disturbances in sleep and appetite, as well as thoughts of death and suicide. As with functional depression, we have identified clinical subtypes, such as major and minor depression. The diagnosis of post-stroke major depression is based on the existence of symptoms of major depression using DSM-III or DSM-IV criteria (American Psychiatric Association, 1980, 1994). The diagnosis of post-stroke minor depression is based on the presence of dysthymic depression using DSM-III criteria or minor depression using DSM-IV criteria (Lipsey et al., 1986). The 2-year duration of symptoms for the diagnosis of dysthymic depression, however, is not required for the diagnosis of minor depression. Symptoms of both subtypes are listed in Table 3.1.

The assessment of symptoms and the diagnosis of depression can be difficult sometimes in stroke patients. For instance, in some patients, the process of clinical interview can be hampered by aphasia. In fact, patients with aphasia involving moderate-to-severe comprehension deficits cannot be reliably diagnosed, because the diagnosis of depression depends upon the patients' ability to understand questions related to their feelings of sadness, hopelessness, and so on. Thus, we have had to exclude such patients from our studies. Finding reliable methods to determine the existence of depression in patients with comprehension and expression impairments is one of the most important problems in the assessment of patients with

Table 3.1

CLINICAL SYNDROME ASSOCIATED WITH CEREBROVASCULAR DISEASE

	Major depression (N=41)	Percent with symptom	Dysthymic depression (N=14)	Percent with symptom
Clinical Symptoms	Depressed mood	100%	Depressed mood	100%
	Diurnal mood variation	76	Anxiety, restlessness, worry	67
	Loss of energy	73	Diurnal mood variation	46
	Anxiety, restlessness, worry	73	Hopelessness	46
	Weight loss, decreased appetite	63	Loss of energy	43
	Early morning awakening	56	Delayed sleep onset	33
	Delayed sleep onset	56	Early morning awakening	26
	Social withdrawal	54	Social withdrawal	23
	Irritability	54	Weight loss, decreased appetite	15
Associated Lesion Location	Left frontal lobe		Right or left posterior parietal and occipital regions	

Source: Robinson, R. G. , Lipsey, J. R., & Price, T. R. (1985). Diagnosis and clinical management of post-stroke depression. *Psychosomatics, 26*, 769-778.

stroke. Also, physical symptoms of depression, such as disturbances of sleep and appetite as well as loss of libido, may occur in medically ill patients as a result of the illness itself, rather than as a concomitant feature of the depression. In cases where a reliable diagnosis cannot be ensured for various reasons, it may be useful to observe the patients for behavioral manifestations of depression and, in some circumstances, to initiate a therapeutic trial of antidepressant medication to see if improvement of these physical symptoms occurs.

DURATION

Based on a 2-year longitudinal study of post-stroke depression, the untreated course of post-stroke major depression is approximately 1 year in duration (Robinson, Bolduc, & Price, 1986). Morris, Robinson, and Raphael (1990) reported a mean duration of 39±31SD weeks for 14 major depression patients. Patients with minor depression, however, appear to have a more variable course. Our studies found that 1 of 10 patients with minor depression in-hospital had major or minor depression 2 years later (Robinson, et al., 1986). Morris and colleagues (1990), however, found the mean duration of minor depression was 12±18SD weeks.

The duration of post-stroke depression is related not only to the clinical subtype of depression but also to the area of brain affected. For instance, we found hemispheric infarcts (i.e., infarcts in the distribution of the middle cerebral artery) result in longer-lasting depression than those involving the brain stem or cerebellum (i.e., in the distribution of the posterior circulation) (Starkstein et al., 1988). Whereas 80% of patients with depressions following hemispheric infarcts (primarily involving the left frontal cortex or left basal ganglia) remained depressed at 6-month follow-up, only 20% of patients with major depressions following brain stem/cerebellar infarcts were still depressed at 6-month follow-up (Robinson et al., 1986). Such differences in duration of depression presumably reflect differences in underlying etiologies and mechanisms.

Thus, post-stroke depression is not a unitary phenomenon. We have identified two (and presumably there are others) of the factors that influence the course of post-stroke depression, depressive diagnosis and lesion location.

RELATIONSHIP OF DEPRESSION TO ASSOCIATED VARIABLES

Lesion Location:

We have consistently found a strong association between the frequency and severity of post-stroke depression and the location of brain injury. Major depression occurs most frequently among patients with left frontal cortex and basal ganglia lesions (Starkstein, Robinson, & Price, 1987). In addition, the severity of depression, as measured by depression rating scales, is directly proportional to the proximity of the anterior border of the lesion to the left frontal pole. This significant linear correlation has held true not only for patients with single lesions of the cortex (Robinson, Kubos, & Starr, 1984; Starkstein et al., 1987), but also for those with bilateral hemispheric lesions (Lipsey et al., 1983), subcortical lesions (Starkstein et al., 1987), and those who are left-handed (Robinson et al., 1985a). In a recent study, we also reported subcortical atrophy, as evidenced by increased ventricle-to-brain ratios, may be an important predisposing factor in the genesis of post-stroke major depression (Starkstein et al., 1988).

Physical Impairment:

The relationship between physical impairment and post-stroke depression is relatively weak compared with the relationship between depression and lesion location. For instance, based on the correlation coefficient between depression severity scores and physical impairment scores, as measured by an activities of daily living scale, physical impairment may account for only 10% of the variance in depression scores, whereas lesion location may account for up to 50% (Robinson et al., 1984). In addition, the cause-and-effect nature of the relationship between depression and physical impairment is uncertain. For example, although one might expect that severe physical impairment would lead to the development of depression, one of our studies found that patients who were depressed (major or minor) in-hospital had greater physical impairment than nondepressed patients with comparable impairments when both groups were followed-up 2 years later (Parikh et al., 1990).

In another study of prognostic indicators related to outcome following stroke, we found severity of in-hospital depression predicted impairment in activities of daily living at 2 years follow-up. In contrast, in-hospital impairment in activities of daily living did not predict severity of depression at 2 years follow-up (Parikh et al., 1988a). Moreover, the disparity in recovery profile between depressed and nondepressed patients is manifest at 2 years follow-up even though the depression has been alleviated in the great majority of cases (Parikh et al., 1990). We have suggested that impaired recovery in activities of daily living may be due to a lack of motivation and initiative to participate in rehabilitative measures, and once the opportunity for early recovery is lost, long-term repercussions in physical recovery may result. In conclusion, the available data suggest that once depression occurs, it interacts with physical impairment. Thus, the most depressed patients remain the most impaired and vice versa (Parikh et al., 1987).

Intellectual Impairment:

The relationship between intellectual impairment and depression is also relatively weak compared with the relationship between depression and lesion location. As physical impairment does not seem to cause depression but instead interacts with it, so also intellectual impairment does not seem to cause depression. Once depression exists, however, it may have a negative impact on intellectual functioning. Evidence suggests that post-stroke major depression may produce a "pseudodementia" or dementia of depression (Bolla-Wilson , Robinson, Starkstein, Boston, & Price, 1989; Starkstein et al., 1988). Thus, patients with major depression perform significantly worse on cognitive tasks than do nondepressed stroke patients who have the same size and location of brain injury (Starkstein et al., 1988). Additionally, the association of cognitive impairment with post-stroke depression occurs only in patients with major depression following *left* hemisphere stroke (Bolla-Wilson et al., 1989; Downhill & Robinson, 1994). The intellectual impairment associated with major depression and left hemisphere stroke is most prominent during the initial in-hospital evaluation but is also demonstrable at 3, 6, and 12 months post-stroke (Downhill & Robinson, 1994). At 2 years post-stroke, no demonstrable association exists between major depression and cognitive impairment (Downhill & Robinson, 1994). House, Dennis, Warlow, Hawton, and Molyneaux (1990) also found that at 1 month following stroke, patients with major depression had significantly more cognitive impairment than patients without a diagnosis.

Social Functioning:

Whereas the degree of premorbid social impairment does not influence the occurrence of post-stroke depression, the severity of depression significantly impacts the social functioning of patients during the recovery period (Robinson et al., 1985b). Patients with the most severe in-hospital depression have the most impaired social functioning at 6-month follow-up. Feibel and Springer (1982) reported significantly more depressed patients had reduced social activities than did nondepressed patients when seen 6 months after their stroke.

REHABILITATIVE TREATMENT

Post-stroke depression is amenable to therapeutic intervention.

A double-blind treatment study conducted at our center with the tricyclic antidepressant nortriptyline (Pamelor) showed that medication to be significantly superior to placebo in alleviating the symptoms of post-stroke depression (Lipsey et al., 1984).

Recently, Andersen, Vestergaard, and Lauritzen (1994) reported the efficacy of the selective serotonin reuptake inhibitor citalopram (10-40 mg/day) in the double-blind treatment of depression in 66 patients who were 2 to 3 months post-stroke. Using either intention to treat (all patients) or efficacy (study completers) analysis, the active-treatment patients showed more improvement in their Hamilton Depression scores over 6 weeks than did placebo-treated controls. Reding et al. (1986) also reported the results of a double-blind treatment study which showed greater improvement in physical functioning in patients who were treated with trazodone (Desyrel) than in patients who received placebo. The interesting implication of this study is that treating post-stroke depression helps alleviate not only the emotional plight of stroke victims, but also helps to improve the process of physical recovery. These findings support our earlier-cited studies that demonstrated the significantly negative impact of post-stroke depression on long-term physical recovery (Parikh et al., 1988a, 1990). It is, therefore, important to recognize and treat post-stroke depression in the early stages.

Our current approach to the rehabilitative management of post-stroke depression consists of accurate diagnosis, careful use of medication, and counseling. The diagnosis of post-stroke depression is confirmed with a thorough clinical examination that assesses patients for affective, cognitive, and behavioral manifestations of depression. Patients with depression then begin treatment with nortriptyline, regardless of the site of the lesion. We generally use nortriptyline in light of our experience and familiarity with that particular tricyclic, but the selective serotonin reuptake inhibitors (SSRIs) have also been demonstrated to be effective. Nortriptyline is the least likely of the tricyclic antidepressants to cause orthostatic hypotension, and it usually has only mild anticholinergic and sedative side effects. Nortriptyline also has a well-documented range of therapeutic serum levels, which is important because some patients — particularly the elderly — may develop higher-than-usual blood levels on a given dosage. In order to minimize the orthostatic or sedative effects of nortriptyline, we administer the full daily dose at bedtime.

We obtain pretreatment electrocardiograms on patients to check for relative contraindications to the drug, which include recent myocardial infarction or significant cardiac conduction anomalies. We also check for narrow-angle glaucoma and urinary tract obstruction. Nortriptyline can potentiate the effects of quinidine and procainamide (Procan) and may prolong the effect of warfarin (Coumadin). Poorly controlled seizure disorders may also be exacerbated. In our treatment study, three patients developed delirious states while on active medication, but, in all three, delirium was reversed when the medication was discontinued. Most patients can be safely treated, therefore, with careful monitoring of the serum levels and side effects. Moreover, untreated depression can be life-threatening. Although the cause of most deaths could not be determined, a 10-year follow-up study of our patients found that the risk of death was 3.5 times greater in patients with in-hospital major or minor depression than similar nondepressed patients with stroke (Morris, Robinson, Andrezejewski, Samuels, & Price, 1993).

We begin most patients on 25 mg of nortriptyline at bedtime for 1 week and then increase the dose to 50 mg for another week. After a week at 50 mg, we obtain a serum level. The serum level is checked earlier if the possibility or presence of side effects is observed. Further dosage adjustments are determined by the serum levels. We attempt to get most patients to the midpoint of the normal therapeutic range, which is between 50 and 150 ng/mL. Most patients require between 50 and 100 mg a day to reach that level. Nortriptyline is one of the few drugs with a documented therapeutic window, so over-shooting the upper limits of the therapeutic range may actually cause worsening of depression. However, it should be remembered that serum levels are a useful, but not necessarily precise, guide to therapeutic monitoring. Clinical response is the ultimate measure of appropriate therapeutic dosage.

Most patients respond within 2–4 weeks after reaching adequate dosage, though some may require up to 6 weeks of treatment. We do not usually consider treatment to be a failure until the patient has been on the therapeutic dosage for at least 6 weeks. Successfully treated patients should be maintained on medication for at least 6 months before a gradual tapering of the medication is attempted. Treatment may be reinstituted if any incipient signs of depression recurrence are present.

Patients who fail to tolerate nortriptyline may be treated with desipramine (Norpramin) or other new generation antidepressants. Nonresponders may be given a therapeutic trial with monoamine oxidase inhibitors or methylphenidate (Ritalin). Other rehabilitative treatment modalities, such as electroconvulsive therapy, family therapy, and group therapy, have also been reported efficacious in managing post-stroke depression (Murray, Shea, & Conn, 1987; Oradei & Waite, 1974; Watzlawick & Coyne, 1980). However, they have not been assessed using control double-blind methodologies.

In addition to treating the depression, the rehabilitation practitioner often needs to help the patient and the family cope with frustrations they may experience during the patient's physical recovery. Sometimes, patients, as well as their relatives, set unrealistically high goals for physical recovery. The rehabilitation specialist must assume an active role in the process of psychosocial assessment of both the patient's inner emotional state and his or her home environment. The vast majority of stroke patients are relieved to have their depression recognized and willingly participate in the treatment process. Despite the availability of literature on the prevalence, severity, and effects of post-stroke depression, as well as research on the efficacy of treatment, many studies indicate the majority of stroke patients do not have their depression recognized and fail to receive treatment of their depression (Collin et al., 1987; Schubert, Taylor, Lee, Mentari, & Tamaklo, 1992). Feibel and Springer (1982) referred to such therapeutic neglect as one of the "great unmet needs of stroke patients."

FUTURE DIRECTIONS

Ultimately, additional studies are needed to address the heterogeneity of the mechanisms and etiologies of depression in patients with stroke. Not all post-stroke depression is the same, and we will not have truly rational treatments until we understand the mechanisms of this disorder. Recent advances in sophisticated neuroimaging techniques, such as positron emission tomography (PET scan) and magnetic resonance imaging (MRI), may facilitate this process. Our studies with PET scanning indicate that a lateralized effect of stroke on serotonin (S2) receptors may play a role in the development of post-stroke depression (Mayberg et al., 1988).

The use of appropriate animal models could also permit a more rigorous and controlled study than is possible in human studies of various neurochemical and neurophysiologic alterations induced by stroke. Data from our model of stroke in the rat indicate a lateralized neurochemical and behavioral effect of stroke and important parallels between the effects of stroke in the rat brain and in the human brain (Robinson, 1979; Parikh et al., 1988b).

The efficacy of various types of treatments of post-stroke depression is another possible productive area for future studies. In particular, the impact of treatment of depression on the intellectual and physical recovery and social functioning of patients with stroke merits greater exploration. Finally, we hope use of the lesion technique in investigating cerebral mechanisms of mood disorders may help clarify the relationship(s) between focal brain areas and specific mood disorders and ultimately expand our knowledge about the mechanisms of normal mood regulation.

REFERENCES

Adams, R. D., & Victor, M. (1985). Cerebrovascular disease. In *Principles of neurology* (pp. 569-640). New York: McGraw-Hill.

American Psychiatric Association. (1980). *Diagnostic and statistical manual of mental disorders* (3rd ed.). Washington, DC: Author.

American Psychiatric Association. (1994). *Diagnostic and statistical manual of mental disorders* (4th ed.). Washington, DC: Author.

Andersen, G., Vestergaard, K., & Lauritzen, L. (1994). Effective treatment of post-stroke depression with the selective serotonin reuptake inhibitor citalopram. *Stroke, 25,* 1099-1104.

Bleuler, E. P. (1951). *Textbook of psychiatry* (pp. 132-197). New York: Macmillan.

Bolla-Wilson, K., Robinson, R. G., Starkstein, S. E., Boston, J., & Price, T. R. (1989). Lateralization of dementia of depression in stroke patients. *American Journal of Psychiatry, 146,* 627-634.

Collin, S. J., Tinson, O., & Lincoln, N. B. (1987). Depression after stroke. *Clinical Rehabilitation, 1,* 27-32.

Downhill, J. E., Jr., & Robinson, R. G. (1994). Longitudinal assessment of depression and cognitive impairment following stroke. *Journal of Nervous and Mental Disease, 182,* 425-431.

Ebrahim, S., Baser, D., & Norin, F. (1987). Affective illness after stroke. *British Journal of Psychiatry, 151,* 52-56.

Feibel, J. H., & Springer, C. J. (1982). Depression and failure to resume social activities after stroke. *Archives of Physical Medicine and Rehabilitation, 63,* 276-278.

Finkelstein, S., Benowitz, L. I., & Baldessarini, R. J. (1982). Mood, vegetative disturbance, and dexamethasone suppression test after stroke. *Annals of Neurology, 12,* 463-468.

Fisher, S. H. (1961). Psychiatric considerations of cerebral vascular disease. *American Journal of Cardiology, 7,* 379-385.

Folstein, M. F., & Maiberger R. (1977). Mood disorders as a specific complication of stroke. *Journal of Neurology, Neurosurgery and Psychiatry, 40*, 1018-1020.

Haroon, E. A. (1986). Psychiatric disturbances following stroke. *Indian Journal of Psychiatry, 28*, 335-341.

House, A., Dennis, M., Warlow, C., Hawton, K., & Molyneaux, A. (1990). The relationship between intellectual and mood disorder in the first year after stroke. *Psychological Medicine, 20*, 805-814.

House, A., Dennis, M., Mogridge, L., Warlow, K., & Jones, L. (1991). Mood disorders the year after stroke. *British Journal of Psychiatry, 158*, 83-92.

Kraepelin, E. (1921). *Manic depressive insanity and paranoia.* Edinburgh: E. & S. Livingstone.

Lipsey, J. R., et al. (1983). Mood change following bilateral hemisphere brain injury. *British Journal of Psychiatry, 143*, 266-273.

Lipsey, J. R., et al. (1984). Nortriptyline treatment of post-stroke depression: A double-blind study. *Lancet, I*, 297-300.

Lipsey, J. R., et al. (1986). Phenomenological comparison of functional and post-stroke depression. *American Journal of Psychiatry, 143*, 527-529.

Mayberg, H., et al. (1988). Pet-imaging of cortical S2 serotonin receptors following stroke: Lateralized changes and relationship to depression. *American Journal of Psychiatry.*

Meyer, A. (1904). The anatomical facts and clinical varieties of traumatic insanity. *American Journal of Insanity, 60*, 373.

Morris, P. L. P., Robinson, R. G., & Raphael, B. (1990). Prevalence and course of depressive disorders in hospitalized stroke patients. *International Journal of Psychiatry in Medicine, 20*, 349-364.

Morris, P. L. P., Robinson, R. G., Andrezejewski, P., Samuels, J., & Price, T. R. (1993). Association of depression with 10-year post-stroke mortality. *American Journal of Psychiatry, 150*, 124-129.

Murray, G. B., Shea, V., & Conn, D. K. (1987). Electroconvulsive therapy for post-stroke depression. *Journal of Clinical Psychiatry, 47,* 258-260.

Oradei, D. M., & Waite, D. S. (1974). Group psychotherapy with stroke patients during the immediate recovery phase. *American Journal of Orthopsychiatry, 44,* 386-395.

Parikh, R. M., et al. (1987). A two-year longitudinal study of post-stroke mood disorders: Dynamic changes in correlates of depression at one and two years follow-up. *Stroke, 18,* 579-584.

Parikh, R. M., et al. (1988a). A two-year longitudinal study of post-stroke mood disorders: Prognostic factors related to one- and two-year outcome. *International Journal of Psychiatry in Medicine, 18,* 45-55.

Parikh, R. M., et al. (1988b). Lateralized effect of cerebral infarction in spinal fluid monoamine metabolite concentrations in the rat. *Stroke, 19,* 472-475.

Parikh, R. M., Robinson, R. G., Lipsey, J. R., Starkstein, S. E., Fedoroff, J. P., & Price, T. R. (1990). The impact of post-stroke depression on recovery in activities of daily living over two-year follow-up. *Archives of Neurology, 47,* 785-789.

Reding, M. J., et al. (1986). Antidepressant therapy after stroke. *Archives of Neurology, 43,* 763-765.

Robinson, R. G. (1979). Differential behavioral and biochemical effects of right and left hemispheric cerebral infarction in the rat. *Science, 205,* 707-710.

Robinson, R. G., et al. (1983). A two-year longitudinal study of post-stroke mood disorders: Findings during the initial evaluation. *Stroke, 14,* 736-741.

Robinson, R. G., et al. (1985a). Mood disorders in left-handed stroke patients. *American Journal of Psychiatry, 142,* 1424-1429.

Robinson, R. G., et al. (1985b). Social functioning assessment in stroke patients: Responses of patients and other informants and relationship of initial evaluation to six months follow-up. *Archives of Physical Medicine and Rehabilitation, 66,* 496-500.

Robinson, R. G., Bolduc, P., & Price, T. R. (1986). A two-year longitudinal study of post-stroke depression: Diagnosis and outcome at one- and two-year follow-up. *Stroke, 18*, 837-843.

Robinson, R. G., Kubos, K. L., & Starr, L. B. (1984). Mood disorders in stroke patients: Importance of location of lesion. *Brain, 107*, 81-93.

Robinson, R. G., & Price, T. R. (1982). Post-stroke depressive disorders: A follow-up study of 103 patients. *Stroke, 13*, 635-641.

Roth, M. (1955). *The natural history of mental disorder in old age* (Maudsley Monograph No. 10). London: Oxford University Press.

Schubert, D. S. P., Taylor, C., Lee, S., Mentari, A., & Tamaklo, W. (1992). Detection of depression in the stroke patient. *Psychosomatics, 33*, 1-5.

Sinyor, D., et al., (1986). Post-stroke depression: Relationship to functional impairment, coping strategies, and rehabilitation outcome. *Stroke, 17*, 1102-1107.

Starkstein, S. E., et al., (1988). Depressive disorders following posterior circulation compared with middle cerebral artery infarcts. *Brain, 111*, 375-387.

Starkstein, S. E., Robinson, R. G., & Price, T. R. (1987). Comparison of cortical and subcortical lesions in the production of post-stroke mood disorders. *Brain, 110*, 1045-1059.

Starkstein, S. E., Robinson, R. G., & Price, T. R. (1988). Comparison of patients with and without post-stroke major depression matched for size and location of lesion. *Archives of General Psychiatry, 45*, 247-252.

Wade, D. T., Legh-Smith, J., & Hewer, R. A. (1987). Depressed mood after stroke, a community study of its frequency. *British Journal of Psychiatry, 151*, 200-205.

Watzlawick, P., & Coyne, J. C. (1980). Depression following stroke: Brief problem-focused family treatment. *Family Process, 19*, 13-18.

4

Anorexia Nervosa, Bulimia Nervosa, and Depression: Multiple Interactions

Arnold E. Andersen, MD

Dr. Andersen is Professor of Psychiatry, The University of Iowa College of Medicine, Iowa City, IA.

KEY POINTS

- It is important to determine the causal relationship between eating disorders and mood disorders in order to grasp the implications for treatment.

- Four interactions between anorexia nervosa and depressive symptoms have been noted. Most significant, there is an increased incidence of mood disorder in the relatives of clients with anorexia nervosa.

- Multiple kinds of interactions also occur between bulimic symptoms and mood disorders. Depression in bulimic clients, often uncovered by clinicians, may lead to alternative mechanisms of unhealthy mood regulation, such as alcohol abuse, drug abuse, or self-injury.

- In the treatment of anorexia nervosa, the goal of therapy is to make the disorder unnecessary rather than take it away. Thus, the encouragement of normal growth and development is especially crucial.

- In the treatment of bulimia nervosa, clients work to find specific methods to deal with the dysphoric mood that produces the need for a "food fix."

- The practicing clinician should avoid a single view of the relationship between eating disorders and mood disorders and instead appreciate the complex, multiple, possible interactions in order to provide a better treatment program.

INTRODUCTION

How are eating disorders and mood disorders related? Are anorexia nervosa and bulimia nervosa variants of depressive illness? Considerable controversy over these issues exists from both a theoretical perspective and in regard to implications for clinical practice. The following discussion attempts to integrate recent research efforts in this area and to summarize a pragmatic approach to patient care. The first generally accepted report of anorexia nervosa was made by Morton in the late seventeenth century, who described "violent passions of the mind" in his patients. Gull and Lasègue, in almost simultaneous reports in the nineteenth century, initiated the modern era of the understanding of eating disorders with their description of the psychopathology and behavioral characteristics of anorexia nervosa. They, too, remarked on the distressed mental state of their patients (Andersen, 1985a).

The best clinical research on the relationship between starvation and mood derives from the landmark work of Keys and colleagues (1950) in the late 1940s. Incidentally, their study was conducted without specific regard to increasing our understanding of eating disorders. Male conscientious objectors underwent losses of almost 25% of their body weight through semistarvation in a study of the global effects of starvation and subsequent methods of rehabilitation. This study clearly demonstrated that starved human beings become apathetic, anhedonic, and asocial. Until recently, the depressed mood of patients with anorexia nervosa was attributed to the nonspecific consequences of starvation, supported by the work of Keys and colleagues.

The simple picture of starvation as the cause of depressive symptomatology started to unravel when Cantwell and associates (1977) and Gershon and co-workers (1984), among others, found a substantial increase in the incidence of depressive illnesses in the relatives of patients with anorexia nervosa. This raised the question of whether anorexia nervosa was, in fact, a variant of depressive illness. The hypothesis that anorexia nervosa causes depression became reversed, and the idea was advocated that depression causes anorexia nervosa.

Bulimia nervosa was first described less than two decades ago in a subgroup of patients hospitalized for anorexia nervosa. Several investigators observed that approximately 40% of hospitalized patients with anorexia nervosa also suffered from binge eating followed by purging. When this group of starved bulimic patients was investigated, it soon became clear that bulimia nervosa existed not only as a subgroup of anorexia nervosa but also could be found in a large number of persons with normal weight who had never manifested anorexia nervosa. The discovery of increased affective disorders in the families of these patients was noticed, and the hypothesis developed that perhaps bulimia nervosa, as well as anorexia nervosa, was a variant of mood disorder (Hudson, 1984).

Two additional developments furthered the idea that mood disorders cause eating disorders. First, several investigators reported that antidepressants decreased bulimic symptoms, probably independent of their effect on mood. Pope and Hudson (1984) described this antibinge effect using tricyclic antidepressants; Walsh and colleagues (1984) conducted trials with monoamine oxidase inhibitors. Second, a number of investigators looked at the lifetime incidence of mood disorders in patients with anorexia nervosa or bulimia nervosa and found a high incidence in these patients as well as in their relatives.

The controversy is perhaps best appreciated by reading back to back the reports of Johnson-Sabine, Wood, & Wakeling (1984) and Hudson and co-workers (1983). The authors of the former article stated fairly confidently that depressive symptoms in patients with bulimia nervosa are nonspecific consequences of their abnormal behaviors; in the latter article, the authors suggested that mood disorders may be integrally related to eating disorders. The basic questions to be answered are: (a) What is the mood state of patients with eating disorders? (b) What *kinds* of depressive syndromes do they have? (c) What is the *causal* relationship between eating disorders and mood disorders? and (d) What are the *implications* for treatment?

A famous scientist is reported to have said something similar to the following: "Make things as simple as possible but no simpler than they actually are." This remark applies to the interaction between mood disorders and eating disorders. The controversy about which disorder is primary and which is secondary becomes moot when the subject is no longer viewed as an "either-or" issue but rather as a "both-and" situation. In fact, mood disorders and eating disorders are related in a complex, multidirectional way. These relationships are perhaps best discussed separately for each of the conditions, anorexia nervosa and bulimia nervosa.

ANOREXIA NERVOSA, RESTRICTING SUBTYPE

Anorexia nervosa and depressive symptoms have at least four kinds of interactions. The observations of Keys and colleagues (1950) are as valid today as when they were first made. Starved patients do, in fact, go into a depressed mood; there is little emotional expression and remarkably little joy and warmth. They differ, however, from patients with classic mood disorders in that they seldom have true psychomotor retardation, early morning awakening, or delusions of guilt or self-blame. They generally lack the agitated depressive state of the handwringing, melancholic patient. However, they do share other depressive symptoms, such as a low mood and lack of emotional responsiveness.

A second, opposite direction of cause and effect occurs when mood change leads to anorexia nervosa. A depressed mood—although not necessarily a depressive syndrome—often initiates the dieting behavior that leads to anorexia nervosa. Attempts to diet generally begin during a time of personal demoralization and dissatisfaction with body size and shape. This second kind of interrelationship, a depressed mood state as *a cause* for the behavior leading to anorexia nervosa, highlights the fact that abnormal eating behaviors may serve as methods to regulate dysphoric mood state.

A third relationship exists between depression and eating disorders that may be uncovered only during treatment. When anorexia nervosa symptoms serve as an unstable but nonetheless temporarily effective way of dealing with depressive symptoms arising from unresolved developmental crises, inadequate treatments that emphasize weight gain alone will unmask the depressive symptoms. Removal of the anorexic symptoms without resolution of the central psychodynamic conflict may uncover, but not resolve, depressive symptoms.

Fourth, depression may appear during the life of patients with anorexia nervosa without being causally related to anorexia nervosa, because both depressive illness and eating disorders share common predisposing factors of a vulnerable temperament and a genetic contribution.

This fourth kind of interaction raises another fundamental question: Why *is* there an increased incidence of mood disorder in the relatives of patients with anorexia nervosa or bulimia nervosa? The following is our hypothesis based on the evaluation and treatment of several hundred patients using the Johns Hopkins Phipps Psychiatric Service. An increased incidence of mood disorders occurs in relatives of patients with anorexia nervosa for two reasons. First, families with affective spectrum disorder generate an increased frequency of the vulnerable personality that is most-predisposing to the development of anorexia nervosa. The vulnerabilities that are essential requirements for the development of anorexia nervosa include low self-esteem, an obsessional style of dealing with problems, and the incorporation of external sociocultural or familial ideals as a way to gain role definition rather than growth from inner ideals. The second way in which these families contribute to the development of eating disorders is by generating, by definition, a high frequency of dysphoric mood states. Eating disorders may then serve to regulate such depressed moods via the alteration in neurotransmitters that these anorexic behaviors produce, especially by self-starvation. The multiple causal relationships between anorexia nervosa and depressive symptoms are summarized in Table 4.1.

Table 4.1

MULTIPLE RELATIONSHIPS BETWEEN AFFECTIVE DISORDERS AND RESTRICTING SUBTYPE OF ANOREXIA NERVOSA: COMPLEX CAUSE-EFFECT INTERACTIONS

- Depression in anorexia nervosa most frequently occurs *secondary* to the biological change of self-starvation

- Depression may be *primary*, with anorexia nervosa occurring to alleviate the depressive symptoms

- Depression may be *tertiary* and represent a psychodynamic response to increased weight and the loss of a coping mechanism that had been used as a short-term method to deal with developmental crises

- Depression and anorexia nervosa may be *independent* and represent common risk factors: vulnerable personality and genetic loading for depressive mood symptoms

---

BULIMIA NERVOSA

As with anorexia nervosa, multiple interactions occur between bulimic symptoms and mood disorders (Table 4.2). Clinicians who see patients with bulimia nervosa agree that these patients feel out of control and are demoralized by their binge-purge behavior. The fourth edition of the *Diagnostic and Statistical Manual of Mental Disorders* (DSM-IV) (American Psychiatric Association, 1994) noted that disparaging self-criticism and a depressed mood often follow eating binges. Bulimia cannot describe the behavior of jaded Roman gourmands who gorged on course after course and vomited to prepare the way for more food. Persons with bulimia nervosa are enormously distressed by their behavior and very seldom consider it egosyntonic, with depressive symptoms occurring secondary to binge-purge behavior.

Table 4.2

THE RELATIONSHIP BETWEEN DEPRESSIVE SYMPTOMS AND BULIMIA NERVOSA: MULTIPLE POSSIBLE KINDS OF INTERACTION

- Most commonly, depression is *secondary* to feeling out of control and helpless

- Not infrequently, depressive symptoms are *primary* and precipitate bulimic behavior by operant conditioning principles because the binge-purge cycle may temporarily help dysphoric mood states

- A *tertiary* interaction is possible: interrupting bulimic symptoms may uncover a depressive state when a method of mastery, coping, and probably neurotransmitter change is taken away. It may be prevented or treated with appropriate psychotherapeutic, behavioral, and pharmacologic methods

- Common etiologic factors may *independently* produce depressive symptoms during the lifetime of the patient, with a higher probability of cluster B traits than in anorexia nervosa

---

The next type of causal connection occurs when depression causes bulimia nervosa. We noted this by listening to patients treated for mood disorder who told us, after improvement of their depression, that nondisclosed symptoms of bulimia nervosa had also improved along with their mood after they were prescribed tricyclic antidepressants. Careful psychiatric histories of these patients showed that bulimic symptoms often serve to regulate a depressed mood state. Whether this regulation is seen in psychodynamic terms as a mastery technique, in behavioral terms as a coping mechanism, or whether it changes neurotransmitter levels is a matter of conjecture. Probably all these mechanisms occur. The fact is that binge behavior may help elevate low mood, and the behavior is perpetuated by classic operant conditioning techniques.

A concern to psychodynamically oriented practitioners has always been the avoidance of symptom substitution. In treatment of bulimia nervosa, patients whose binge-purge behavior is decreased without attention to the purposes it serves may experience previously hidden depression because their behavioral mechanism of mood regulation has been removed. This uncovered depression may lead to alternative mechanisms of unhealthy mood regulation, such as alcohol abuse, other kinds of drug abuse, or self-injury. Moreover, bulimic patients may have mood disorders independent of their eating disorder because of their vulnerability toward the independent expression of each of these syndromes on the basis of a predisposed temperament and genetic loading. The vulnerable personality in bulimia nervosa may include more self-dramatizing and "borderline" features than in anorexia nervosa, as well as the shared low self-esteem and obsessional style. The multiple interrelationships between bulimic symptoms and depressive symptoms are described in Table 4.2.

ANOREXIA NERVOSA, BULIMIC SUBTYPE

DSM-IV criteria for diagnosis of psychiatric disorders formally divides anorexia nervosa into food restricting and binge/purge subtypes, a practice used informally for a decade by researchers in the United States and clinicians in Europe. Patients with the bulimic subtype of anorexia nervosa suffer from a combination of the self-starvation of restricting anorexia nervosa and the out-of-control distress of bulimia nervosa. They have the highest overall measures of psychological distress and medical symptomatology. Their depressive symptoms represent a combination of features from Tables 4.1 and 4.2.

IMPLICATIONS FOR PRACTICE: ANOREXIA NERVOSA

Our experience suggests that the low mood that accompanies the starvation of anorexia nervosa is best treated by prompt nutritional rehabilitation. Restoration of normal body weight often, but not always, alleviates the anhedonic, depressed mood. If weight restoration and intensive psychotherapy do not improve mood, and if patients still meet DSM-IV criteria for major depressive disorder, vigorous treatment to achieve therapeutic blood levels with tricyclic antidepressants or with standard dosages of selective serotonin reuptake inhibitors (SSRIs) is warranted. Unfortunately, evidence is lacking suggesting that antidepressants are uniformly beneficial for all food-restricting anorectic patients in the starved state unless they have associated symptoms of mood disorder at restored weights. When anorexia nervosa appears to be the result of initial depressive symptoms, rather than the cause of them, antidepressants may be employed sooner in treatment and continued for 6–9 months after weight restoration. We generally start with fluoxetine (Prozac) or paroxetine (Paxil) because of the high safety, moderate side effects, and lack of carbohydrate craving produced. Any of the standard tricyclics may also be used, however. Some advocacy of high-dose SSRIs to improve the central psychopathological symptoms of a morbid fear of fatness and the relentless drive for thinness recently has been made on the basis of open-blind studies; however, convincing evidence of their effectiveness for this purpose is not yet present.

The uncovering of depressive symptoms by a purely behavioral or mechanical approach toward refeeding can be avoided by integrating a comprehensive psychotherapeutic approach toward treatment. This means attending to the psychodynamic aspects of anorexia nervosa, the social and familial consequences of the disorder, and the psychopathological characteristics of fear of fatness, pursuit of slimness, and perceptual distortion. The goal of therapy is to make this disorder unnecessary rather than to take it away (Andersen, 1985b). The goals sought by dieting behavior in patients who develop anorexia nervosa are usually desirable, understandable ones. We tell patients that we endorse their goals, such as feeling better about themselves and being more effective, but ask them to work with us to find more adaptive, less harmful methods to accomplish these goals. This means developing a therapeutic alliance with their observing ego, employing the resources of the healthy, rational part of the self in order to deal with the symptoms and behaviors of the illness. A decrease in symptomatology is only a part of the treatment of anorexia nervosa. The encouragement of normal growth and development, especially the capacity to identify and deal directly with developmental challenges and to experience positive mood states, are major goals of treatment.

Much remains unknown about the long-term consequences of anorexia nervosa. Our observations suggest that when patients do improve, they may remain vulnerable to repeated episodes of the eating disorders and may experience a variety of the syndromes clustered under the term *affective spectrum disorders*, which includes obsessive-compulsive symptoms, frank depressive episodes, dysthymic disorders, and alcoholism. Hall and associates (1984) found that 50% of patients with eating disorders developed another psychiatric syndrome on follow-up. On a more positive note, there is growing evidence that patients may not only "recover," as with addictive disorders, but may be permanently improved after treatment, and in some ways better than if they had never been ill because successful treatment involves coming to terms with profound societal forces interacting with individual development.

IMPLICATIONS FOR TREATMENT: BULIMIA NERVOSA

We employ methods similar but not identical to those used in the treatment of anorexia nervosa in patients suffering from bulimia nervosa. Initial efforts are directed at interrupting the binge-purge behavior to alleviate the demoralization that comes from being out of control. Regular, balanced meals are prescribed, with an adequate intake of complex carbohydrates and low fat protein, and the avoidance of food fads. Weight change is undertaken, if necessary, only slowly, and only after food intake is regular. Psychotherapy begins with supportive and educational methods but soon incorporates cognitive and psychodynamic techniques. Whereas anorexic patients often have difficulty in identifying their mood state, bulimic patients may experience a diffuse dysphoria, which they find intolerable and previously had been alleviated only by binging. Patients work in individual and group therapy to identify specific moods states, to tolerate their presence for reasonable periods without short-circuiting the mood with a "food fix," and to find specific methods to deal with the dysphoric mood that target the symptom or its cause in healthy ways.

The data are not yet clear as to whether antidepressants effectively decrease binge behavior independent of mood state. Somewhat exaggerated claims have been made for their effectiveness, sometimes leading to the prescribing of these medications as the complete treatment of bulimia nervosa. Many patients are relieved of their bulimic behavior by a combination of behavioral methods and cognitive psychotherapy techniques without any medication. When antidepressants are used, they should be employed as part of a comprehensive treatment program that includes psychotherapy and attempts to deal with the social and familial aspects of the illness.

A history of clear, prebulimic depressive episodes initiating binge episodes suggests that long-term treatment with antidepressants may be beneficial. As with any depressive illness, lithium supplementation for augmentation or a switch to newer antidepressants (e.g., venlafaxine [Effexor]) in place of an SSRI or tricyclic may be warranted. Little evidence suggests that the newer antidepressants are clearly superior, but they may produce more tolerable side effects. Documented blood levels within a therapeutic range for 4–6 weeks are usually necessary to make a judgment about the effectiveness of a tricyclic antidepressant, or in the case of SSRIs, 6–8 weeks of standard dosage.

The two major causes of death in patients with eating disorders are starvation and suicide for anorexia nervosa and cardiac disorders and suicide for bulimia nervosa. Clinicians must, therefore, be attentive to mood state and possible suicide in these patients, as in all clients with depressive symptoms (Garner et al., 1984). The more impulsive suicide attempts found in bulimic patients with cluster B personality disorders are harder to predict and may be less responsive to medications.

SUMMARY

Mood symptoms are found in most, if not all, patients with anorexia nervosa and bulimia nervosa. The practicing clinician should avoid taking a single view of the relationship between these disorders and appreciate instead the complex, multiple, possible interactions. Even though anorexia nervosa may have egosyntonic features with a false sense of mastery, it is frequently associated with a lowered mood state, the major contributing feature being the starved state. Bulimia nervosa symptoms are frankly egodystonic in the great majority of patients and a source of demoralization and secondary depression.

Prompt treatment of the underlying starvation in anorexia nervosa and the binge-purge behavior in bulimia nervosa improves mood in a majority of these patients. Where the symptoms have served to regulate dysphoric mood states, direct treatment of the lowered mood with antidepressants as well as psychotherapeutic methods may be helpful. Purely mechanical or strictly behavioral approaches to these disorders may lead to the uncovering of depressive symptoms formerly regulated by the eating disorder. Anticipation of this possible consequence with a comprehensive psychotherapeutic treatment program will often prevent this state of uncovered depression or deal with it as it occurs.

Finally, the factors common to the origin of both eating disorders may lead to independent expression of a variety of syndromes associated with the affective disorders spectrum over the life span of a patient. Ongoing research studies that are exploring the interrelation between mood disorders and eating disorders will lead, hopefully, to an appreciation of the variety of mood states that occur in patients with anorexia nervosa or bulimia nervosa, a better understanding of the affective syndromes to which these mood states belong, and to increasingly effective long-term treatment.

REFERENCES

American Psychiatric Association. (1994). *Diagnostic and statistical manual of mental disorders* (4th ed.). Washington, DC: Author.

Andersen, A. E. (1985a). Three classic papers on anorexia nervosa: The work of Morton, Gull, and Lasègue. In A. E. Andersen (Ed.), *Comprehensive practical treatment of anorexia nervosa and bulimia* (chap. 2, pp. 10–27). Baltimore: Johns Hopkins University Press.

Andersen, A. E. (Ed.) (1985b). *Comprehensive practical treatment of anorexia nervosa and bulimia.* Baltimore: Johns Hopkins University Press.

Cantwell, D. P., et al. (1977). Anorexia nervosa: An affective disorder? *Archives of General Psychiatry, 34,* 1087–1093.

Garner, D. M., et al. (1984). Psychoeducational principles in the treatment of bulimia and anorexia nervosa. In D. M. Garner & P. E. Garfinkel (Eds.), *Handbook of psychotherapy for anorexia nervosa and bulimia.* New York: Guilford Press.

Gershon, E. S., et al. (1984). Clinical findings in patients with anorexia nervosa and affective illness in their relatives. *American Journal of Psychiatry, 141*, 1419–1422.

Hall, A., et al. (1984). Anorexia nervosa: Long-term outcome in 50 female patients. *British Journal of Psychiatry, 145*, 407–413.

Hudson, J. I. (1984). Bulimia: A form of affective disorder? In S. H. Frazier (Ed.), *McLean hospital journal* (chap. IX, pp. 31–45). Belmont, MA: McLean Hospital.

Hudson, J. I., et al. (1983). Phenomenologic relationship of eating disorders to major affective disorder. *Psychiatry Research, 9*, 345-354.

Johnson-Sabine, E. C., Wood, K. H., & Wakeling, A. (1984). Mood changes in bulimia nervosa. *British Journal of Psychiatry, 145*, 512–516.

Keys, A. et al. (1950). *The biology of human starvation* (vol. II). Minneapolis: University of Minnesota Press.

Pope, H. G., & Hudson, J. I. (1984). *New hope for binge eaters.* Cambridge, MA: Harper & Row.

Walsh, B. T., et al. (1984). Treatment of bulimia with phenelzine: A double-blind placebo-controlled study. *Archives of General Psychiatry, 41*, 1105–1109.

5

Group Counseling for Depressed Older Adults

Wanda Y. Johnson, PhD, PC

Dr. Johnson is a Licensed Professional Counselor, Licensed Marriage and Family Therapist, Certified Hypnotherapist, and Certified Play Therapist who has a private practice in Arlington, TX. Her areas of expertise include group psychotherapy and depression.

KEY POINTS

- Current research suggests an increase in the elderly population. This "graying of society" affects us all; it is important to develop sound, specialized clinical skills in counseling older adults.

- Older adults are highly susceptible to depression; however, little research has been conducted on the effect of depression on the elderly.

- Factors that make older adults susceptible to depression include: limited incomes, poor housing, a greater vulnerability to street crime, social isolation, family communication problems, and losses of family members and/or spouses.

- Group therapy with older adults can be extremely effective in treating depression: it affords them a structure within which to offer each other hope and encouragement; gives them a chance to learn about themselves, the aging process, family interactions, and the symptoms and course of depression; and provides them with an opportunity to maintain social interaction and mental activity.

- Various beneficial techniques for working with older adults in a group setting are presented: educational/therapeutic, life review, psychodrama, intergenerational, bereavement, assertiveness training, and exercise.

INTRODUCTION

As our population grows older, few researchers would disagree that improving the quality of life of the elderly warrants much attention. To be sure, better health care for older adults (persons who are older than 65) must be developed. Both their quality of life and general health depend upon the prevention of mental health problems and the treatment of emotional disturbances. Although it is difficult to determine the percentage of older adults suffering from depression, most mental health professionals estimate that depression is quite common in this population (e.g., Papolos & Papolos, 1987).

Population projections suggest both a numerical and proportionate increase in the number of persons in the older age groups. One investigator suggested that by the year 2000, more than 17 million people will be 75 years or older; by the year 2025, this number will exceed 25 million; and the population aged 85 and older, nearly 2.3 million in 1980, is projected to exceed 7 million by the year 2025. The youngest members of the "baby-boom" generation will turn 65 years old by the year 2030 (Brody, 1985).

This "graying" of American society affects all of us and has been the object of much recent attention. Demographic shifts in the general population underscore the importance of developing sound, specialized clinical skills in counseling older adults. Group therapy is one such tool in the mental health professional's therapeutic armamentarium. This chapter, which touches upon the rationale for utilizing groups in treating depression in the elderly, will discuss special counseling concerns of the elderly as well as the nuances of group work in this client population. But, first, we must decide who qualifies as an "older adult" and arrive at a solid understanding of the nature of depression in the elderly.

CATEGORIZING OLDER ADULTS

Gerontologists recognize three types of aging: biologic, psychological, and social. Biologic age refers to how well the physical body systems are working; psychological age is concerned with self-image, self-esteem, adaptive ability, one's worldview, and relationships with others; and social age encompasses the behavioral expectations of persons of a given age. Expectations about an older person's position and status in society, manner of dressing, relationship to children, marital status, and the like are included in social age.

We frequently speak of cohort groups when trying to understand persons of a specific age group. "Cohort" refers to any group of people born within a given year or other specified short period. For example, persons born in 1900, 1920, and 1960 comprise three distinct cohorts. Each cohort group is exposed to a unique set of experiences throughout life. Some of these experiences are shared experiences, such as wars, depressions, and stock market crashes. Other experiences are unique to each person. To understand any cohort of adults, one must understand something about the convergence of historic, social, religious, and economic factors that influenced their lives. The factors determine the social and familial norms for feminine and masculine behavior that prevailed during the formative and subsequent years. A person born in 1920 would have very different experiences from a person born in 1960, yet there undoubtedly would be experiences common to both persons — although they are subject to interpretation through different viewpoints. Counselors must constantly resist the temptation to attribute differences simply to age. Chronologic age is important primarily in identifying the cultural and ideologic factors that may have influenced a person and his or her cohort.

Persons born in different generations have vastly different life experiences. In trying to disentangle the differences among people of different generations, Schaie (1965) made the distinction between age *differences* and age *changes*. Age changes are those aspects of development related to the aging process and can be judged only by following the same person over time. Age differences can be judged by comparing people of different ages.

Recognizing that older adults are more diverse than alike, one should also recognize the broad age span between the ages of 65 and 90. Categorizing these persons as "older people" results in a vastly diverse assortment. Within this age group, there is a multiple variance in mental and physical health, educational experience, personality traits, and interests. The principal behavioral feature of the elderly may be the vast range of abilities found among them. Most research has shown a pattern of increasing statistical variance in the scores of the elderly on psychological measures when compared with those of younger adults. That is, differences among older persons are more vast than those among younger persons. Such differences should not be surprising considering the complex factors that affect human abilities, including genetic endowment, opportunities for learning, and motivation.

Researchers frequently place older adults into two groups: the "young old" — persons between the ages of 65 and 75 — and the "old old" — adults 75 years and older. In a report on aging, the Subcommittee on Human Services of the Select Committee on Aging, U.S. House of Representatives, suggested that there are two natural seasons of life: senior adulthood, ages 60 to 75, and elderhood, 75 years plus. The Committee found that adults in senior adulthood were functionally independent, whereas adults in elderhood were more dependent and more likely to require special care (Nelson, 1982). It remains important to remember that there may be few changes due to aging itself. Although some generalizations may be helpful, others may foster stereotypes that are hindrances to understanding individual adults.

DEPRESSION IN OLDER ADULTS

A major concern regarding the older adult population is the incidence of depression. Papolos and Papolos (1987) estimate that 15%–20% of persons who are 65 years and older suffer from depression. Although the link between depression and death in older adults is unclear, a 9-year follow-up study of

New Haven-area residents interviewed for the Epidemiologic Catchment Area (ECA) study suggested a high death rate among people with certain mental disorders. Both men and women were more likely to die given recent depression, with the odds ratio for men 4.22:1 and the odds ratio for women 1.65:1. These findings raise a question regarding the common belief that the rate of depression has been rising in the past two generations, suggesting that older adults may have a lower-than-average lifetime rate of depression largely because persons susceptible to depression tend to die young (Bruce, Leaf, Rozal, Florio, & Hoff, 1994).

Difficulty of Diagnosis:

One reason for the lack of data on the effect of depression on the elderly is the difficulty of making a definitive diagnosis of depression in this population. In older adults, depressive symptoms often mimic other conditions, such as Alzheimer's disease and dementia. Approximately 12% of older persons diagnosed with dementia actually suffer from a false dementia arising from untreated depression (Papolos & Papolos, 1987). Although treating a patient with Alzheimer's disease for depression can often be beneficial, treating a depressed person for dementia is not beneficial whatsoever.

Dementia and depression also often coexist. In its early stages, dementia can be difficult to distinguish from depression. The term *dementia* actually refers to a group of chronic diseases that are similar in that there is a progressive, often gradual decline in intellectual functions. The onset usually begins with an impairment in memory of relatively recent events. Gradually, abstract reasoning becomes impaired, judgment is affected, and language skills and well-established memory eventually erodes (Zarit, 1980). According to the fourth edition of the *Diagnostic and Statistical Manual of Mental Disorders* (DSM-IV) (American Psychiatric Association, 1994), a diagnosis of dementia is based on a pattern of cognitive deficits and is not necessarily progressive. Indeed, dementia may be progressive, static, or remitting. Based on studies cited in the DSM-IV, 2%–4% of the population suffer from dementia of the Alzheimer's type; other types of dementia are much less common. The prevalence of dementia, especially dementia of the Alzheimer's type and cerebral vascular dementia, increases with age. An increase in the prevalence of dementia occurs after age 75, with a prevalence of 20% or more in persons older than age 85. Direct pathologic diagnosis of dementia of the Alzheimer's type is almost impossible to obtain, so the diagnosis is made by ruling out all other etiologies of the dementia.

The symptoms of depression can often mimic those of dementia. In older adults, depression may cause memory problems, muddle thought processes, and impair concentration. Such vegetative symptoms can create difficulty in taking care of oneself. It is interesting to note that health care professionals in the United States diagnose dementia more frequently than do health care professionals in Britain. British psychiatrists tend to diagnose depression more often when treating older adults and seem to work more actively to help geriatric patients (Belsky, 1984). In working with elderly patients with Alzheimer's disease and/or dementia, the conscientious counselor should consider the possible presence of depression — either in conjunction with or independent of the other two diseases. If depression is found to exist, its proper treatment could prove beneficial to the patient.

Other factors also confound the diagnosis of depression in older adults. Elderly people, who often attend less to changes in mood and attitude, may complain of physical ailments rather than depressive symptoms. Some older adults may appear confused, evidence memory loss, be agitated, and lose interest in life events; nevertheless, they may not attribute these symptoms to depression. Physicians, too, may try to treat these symptoms as indicative of a physical ailment rather than a mood disorder.

In older adults, depressive symptoms may be underreported by patients or may not reach the level of clinical depression, but, of course, they still require treatment. Proper treatment may include both pharmacologic and psychotherapeutic regimens. Often, similar underlying biologic mechanisms may be at work, including degenerative brain changes. In one study, brain scans of depressed patients in their 60s suggested tissue loss in the frontal lobes of the cerebral cortex by comparison with healthy controls the same age ("Update on Mood Disorders," 1994). Fogel (1991) suggested that dopaminergic and noradrenergic reserves may decline in older adults, which may contribute to depressive symptomatology. In such an event, antidepressants may help depressive symptoms even when they are not at the threshold warranting the diagnosis of a clinical depression.

A patient's own lack of cooperation as well as cultural inhibitions can be obstacles in diagnosing depression. Older adults' reluctance to ask for help and to recognize the need for counseling can be a barrier to revealing the information needed for an accurate diagnosis of depression. Some cohorts of older adults perceive the need for counseling very differently from younger cohorts. They are more likely to believe that any mental health problem imposes a stigma. Therefore, they may hide their concerns, report only physical complaints, and refuse to seek counseling. Moreover, older adults may believe the stereotypes and myths about aging and have a fatalistic view of their later years. Their fear of a diagnosis of Alzheimer's disease may lead them to avoid seeking help.

Susceptible Cases:

Some older adults are susceptible to depression simply because their situations are depressing. Such older persons struggling with limited incomes, poor housing, a greater vulnerability to street crime, social isolation, family communication problems, and losses of family members and/or a spouse have an increased susceptibility to depression. In developing the patient history, the prudent counselor should investigate these areas.

White men older than age 65 are particularly vulnerable to

depression. The suicide rate for these men becomes increasingly higher after age 60. By age 85, the suicide rate for white men is three times that of any other population (Miller, 1979). The specific reasons for these deaths are, of course, unknown. However, there is a real possibility that the reversals of old age hit this group harder due to their difficulty in adjusting to changes from a former position of privileged social status.

A possible intervention is group counseling focused on preparation for lifestyle changes. Group counseling can also help older adult men adjust to changes and create support for each other during this critical phase of their lives. Reconstructing the events prior to suicide for a number of older white men, Miller (1979) noted that many of the men who chose suicide visited their family physician shortly before their death. This suggests a possible attempt for assistance from a professional. Unfortunately, most physicians are not trained to ask the proper questions or to recognize the symptoms of the potential suicide.

Adaptation to Loss:

A significant area to explore when counseling older adults is that of "loss," both actual and impending. Adaptation to loss and acceptance of the imminence of one's death may be two of the central tasks of old age. Losses suffered by older adults may be many and varied. The loss of one's abilities, social skills, status, finances, as well as friends, family members, and perhaps a spouse is a difficult adjustment for most people. The elderly may be more vulnerable to the effects of loss than younger persons. Limited opportunities for new involvement with people, or limited psychological capacities, may affect an older adult's ability to compensate for losses.

From a psychological perspective, losses that occur in rapid succession can keep a person in a perpetual state of grieving. If left unresolved, the effect of such losses diminishes the quality of life and perhaps contributes to a depressed state.

A 90-year-old woman, widowed for 40 years and with no living family members, reported that the thing she missed most having was friends and siblings with whom she had a "shared past." "I miss having a sister or brother, a friend, or a husband who laughs at the same things I laugh at. My sister and I used to talk about our childhood and laugh and laugh. Now the same stories are not funny to anyone else."

Such experiences are often responsible for considerable dysfunction in the elderly and, conversely, may be an important springboard for beneficial therapy.

SPECIAL COUNSELING CONCERNS OF OLDER ADULTS

Concern has been expressed within the counseling profession regarding the need for special therapeutic skills in counseling older adults. The threshold question is: "Are the same techniques and skills used with younger adults applicable to working with older adults?" The increase in the number of university courses, special journal issues, counseling divisions, and funding for projects strongly suggests the need for specific preparation for counseling older adults.

Counselors must recognize several basic considerations in dealing with any special population. As always, the first consideration for counselors is to have a thorough understanding of themselves, their responses to the population, and the self-presence of any subtle biases or set of expectations. Second, counselors require pertinent knowledge about the specific population and whether any differences make that population distinct. Finally, they should be skilled in the counseling modalities and techniques found to be most effective in treating that population.

Counselors' views of old age and the changes that accompany aging are important. Some counselors, like the general public, maintain that it is more valuable to treat younger persons. Younger people have their entire lives ahead of them, whereas older people have a shorter life expectancy and, therefore, warrant less attention. Another view holds that older adults simply cannot benefit from psychological adjustment. Both attitudes are erroneous. It is vital for counselors working with older adults to view aging in terms of continued potential for growth rather than in terms of inevitable loss. Counselors interested in treating older adults should complete the self-examination presented in Table 5.1.

CURATIVE INFLUENCES OF GROUP THERAPY

Group therapy has various applications far beyond the treatment of emotionally disturbed persons. Groups are designed to aid in the resolution of a variety of issues, such as adjusting to retirement, overcoming stress, changing sexual attitudes, combating bias, modifying Type-A behavior, adjusting to family transitions, enhancing careers, and adapting to a nursing home. Although psychotherapy groups are distinctive in that they are designed to help clients with emotional problems resolve their difficulties, many groups have psychotherapeutic components.

Yalom (1975) described a series of curative influences involved in therapy groups. Groups aid interpersonal learning and allow group members to develop socializing techniques. Honest responses from group members enable members to see the impact of their communication style and behavior upon others. Members can practice new communication skills and behavior in the safety of the group setting.

Groups also foster positive change by offering mutual support and normalizing problems because of the insight that many people may share the same problems. This is extremely important, for example, because one element of depression is an overwhelming sense of isolation. The discovery (through sharing of experiences and feelings in a group setting) that others have the same problems, doubts, and fears can be a tremendous healing revelation.

Group counseling affords older adults the opportunity to

Table 5.1
SELF-EXAMINATION FOR COUNSELORS INTERESTED IN TREATING
OLDER ADULTS

1. What are my opinions about old people?
2. What do I believe about aging?
3. What understanding do I have about the specific elderly cohorts with whom I am working?
4. Do I have fears about aging or elderly persons?
5. Do I treat elderly people as if they are frail?
6. Can I value an elderly person?
7. Do I have a history of positive experiences with older people?
8. Do I enjoy interacting with elderly people?
9. Do I have an understanding of the effect of life experiences on the communication patterns of older adults?
10. Am I patient with persons who have physical disabilities?
11. Am I comfortable with grief?
12. Am I sensitive to the social, cultural, and economic influences upon the elderly?
13. Do I have a solid background in the physical aspects of aging?
14. Do I have knowledge of the special biologic, psychological, and social needs of the elderly?
15. Do I believe in the worth of therapy for the elderly?
16. Can I challenge the myths about aging?
17. Can I comfortably confront mistaken beliefs, irrational beliefs, and ineffective communication styles when manifested in the elderly?
18. Do I thoroughly understand the difference between dementia and depression?
19. Do I have unresolved issues with my parents or grandparents?
20. Do I believe that therapy for older people can help to modify the maladaptive attitudes, self-defeating behavior, and upsetting feelings limiting their lives?
21. Do I believe that group therapy is an effective technique for older adults?
22. Do I believe that mental health intervention for the elderly is an important allocation of services for society?

encourage each other and offer hope that change is possible. For older adults, an important benefit of group counseling is the chance to offset some of the loss and loneliness they feel. This therapeutic modality provides an opportunity to maintain mental activity and social interaction, as members can watch and learn from each other. In counseling groups, older adults have the chance to help one another by acting as therapists for one another while sharing insights and support.

These benefits strongly suggest that group therapy with older adults can be particularly effective. Psychotherapy groups have been formed to help a variety of elderly persons, ranging from the minimally impaired to severely impaired (Zarit, 1980).

THE DYNAMICS OF ELDERLY GROUPS

Counseling groups can be expressly designed to treat depression with a variety of techniques. Exercise groups, groups designed to inform members about depressive symptoms, assertiveness groups — as well as any group that provides a forum for interaction, exchange of thoughts and feelings and introspection — can be worthwhile endeavors for older adults suffering from depression.

Member Selection:

As with any group, the purpose, goals, and techniques used in the group must be clearly delineated; this information should be provided to potential group members. According to the *Ethical Guidelines for Group Counselors* (Association for Group Work, 1990), prospective group members should have access to the information presented in Table 5.2. The prudent counselor will provide this information to each member of the group in writing for the protection of both the member and the counselor.

Selection and preparation of members for the group require

forethought. For elderly groups, selecting members who can both benefit from the group experience and contribute to the group experience is especially important. Counselors must carefully investigate potential group members for any individual impairment. Combining persons who function at a high level with those who may be severely impaired negates the benefit of group therapy. Counselors' judgment in selecting members for the group should be combined with a clear explanation of the group's composition to prospective members.

Table 5.2
INFORMATION FOR PROSPECTIVE GROUP MEMBERS

1. A statement of the goals and purposes of the group
2. Entrance procedures, time limits of the group experience, and termination procedures
3. The rights and responsibilities of both group members and the group leader
4. The techniques and procedures that may be used, especially any specialized or experimental activities in which members may be expected to participate
5. The education, training, and qualifications of the group leader
6. The fees and any other related expenses
7. A statement of whether follow-up services are included in the fee
8. A realistic statement of what services will and will not be provided within a particular group structure
9. The personal risks, if any, involved in the group
10. The use of, or prohibition against, any recording of the sessions
11. Confidentiality expectations and limitations

Adapted from: Ethical Guidelines for Group Counselors (Association for Group Work, 1990), pp. 119-126. Copyright ACA. Reprinted with permission. No further reproduction authorized without written permission of the American Counseling Association.

Groups composed of persons both older and younger than age 65 can be very effective, and all participants can benefit greatly from learning about perceptions from one another. In

conducting multifamily, weekend groups of patients hospitalized for treatment of depression, I have found the combination
of older and younger clients to be mutually therapeutic. The
age of the group members frequently ranged from 18 years to
the late 60s. Patients' insights into family interactions are often
more easily absorbed while hearing and watching members of
other families talk about their feelings. Moreover, effective
resolution of intergenerational family differences may occur,
even among patients with no family members present.

Decisions on whether to limit groups to same-sex members
or to include both sexes may affect group functioning. Statistically, because of the longevity differences between men and
women, fewer men are available for group inclusion than
women. Some studies show that women share more readily
with each other more often in all-women groups, whereas in
mixed-gender groups, women seem to have minimal contact
with each other and allow men to dominate the group discussion (Aries, 1976); this holds true more often for older than
younger cohorts of adults. Women in mixed-gender groups
tend not to assert themselves or assume leadership.

Another decision revolves around the benefit of including
some married couples in groups with single clients. The advantages of inclusion should be carefully considered and
discussed with group members.

Special Concerns:

For older adults, smaller sized groups of four to eight
members may be more beneficial than larger groups. (The
smaller sized group is less threatening.) It is also easier for
adults with visual or hearing impairments to participate in
smaller groups. If physical ailments create a low energy level,
smaller groups allow time for everyone in the group to participate.

Vision and hearing loss should be expected by group therapists. The group room should be well lit, with glare minimized

and extraneous background noise eliminated if possible. Group members should be encouraged to speak out when they have trouble seeing or hearing so that compensations can be made. The energy level of physically impaired older persons must also be addressed. The proposed length of each group meeting should be discussed with the participants so an optimum time can be established.

PHASES OF GROUP DEVELOPMENT

The Initial Phase:

The initial phase of group work with older adults may take longer than that in groups composed of younger clients. Counselors must exercise patience and sensitivity. Group cohesiveness in older groups may evolve somewhat differently from other groups. In part, this is due to the difficulty in forming new friendships, a common problem with older adults. This becomes a crucial problem for the older adult who moves into a new community, retirement center, or nursing home. Because we become more different than alike as we age, it is sometimes difficult to find adults with common interests. In addition, older adults report that it takes too much energy to form new friendships and that they are reluctant to become close to people because of all the pain from prior losses of friends and family members.

With a group of older people who are psychologically unaware, and perhaps reluctant to talk about personal matters with others, their ability to talk about their feelings or family life in a group may initially be inhibited. More time and initial training in communication skills are needed with elderly groups than with groups of younger adults. As with all groups, clearly defined group goals and a delineated group structure are essential.

The leader can help members become comfortable by actively teaching listening and responding skills and exploring how to show understanding without agreement. Often, members should be taught how to say "no" to each other and how to ask for more time to discuss emotional issues. It is also important to allow time for members to become comfortable in the group and for the leader to show patience and understanding during the initial phase. Finally, group leaders need to demonstrate and model respect for members' decision to proceed at their own pace.

Initially, discussion may focus on philosophical aspects of aging, general life concerns, current events, or even favorite television shows and books. The group may be more comfortable offering advice than empathizing with each other. Some group leaders report that sharing their own self-revelations is helpful in facilitating self-revelations by group members. Encouragement and modeling by counselors may be necessary to facilitate members' talking about and among themselves. It is difficult to discern whether reticence stems from any possible rugged individualism and self-control characteristics of a specific cohort, the current living situation, or the aging process.

The Active Phase:

As the anxiety and unease of revealing feelings subside, the group becomes more cohesive and supportive. Discussion can then center on personal feelings and "here-and-now" issues. Members may begin working through some of their cognitions, feelings, and perceptions of past experiences. They can support each other in enjoying life and planning for the future. Sometimes, the fresh perspective of others can reframe old beliefs and can allow members to release feelings of guilt and self-recrimination in favor of self-acceptance.

The group leader may find the need to structure elderly groups more than groups of adolescents or younger adults. The structure may take the form of introducing topics for discussion each session and explaining what needs to be accomplished during that session.

The Termination Phase:

The termination phase of a group may be especially difficult for older adults because of the accumulation of losses suffered during their lives. Once a member has accepted the group process, he or she may view the termination of the group as another loss. Therefore, group termination should be planned and ample time allowed to process feelings and encourage the formation of additional support groups and the continuation of friendships formed through the group. Counselors can facilitate continued social interactions by pointing out the advantages of alliances and noting the behavior that simplifies friendship formation and communication. Adequate preparation for leaving the group will inoculate group members against the depression that sometimes follows termination of a group.

TYPES OF ELDERLY GROUPS

Group treatment of depression in older adults can focus on the differences in this population. Depression may be the center of treatment *per se* or can be addressed as part of a broader program. Symptoms of depression can be treated through a variety of groups and techniques. Counselors may prevent depressive symptoms from becoming debilitating by educating older adults and helping them undertake behavioral changes that enhance their quality of life. Groups combining an educational component with time for group interaction and interpretation seem to work optimally.

Helping older adults build (or regain) a sense of self-worth and appreciate their strengths are important therapeutic goals for groups dealing with depression. Groups that help older adults to learn about themselves, the aging process, family interactions over their life span, and the symptoms and course of depression go a long way in alleviating depression. The focus should be placed on the behavioral regimen needed to combat depressive symptomatology.

Educational/Therapeutic:

Combining educational and therapeutic components into group work is a useful design when working with older adults. Recent interest in elder hostels on college campuses attests to older adults' eagerness to continue learning late in life. Such learning has long been recognized as a deterrent to depression, and research now suggests that lifelong learning or regular mental exercise can prevent — or at least delay — the onset of Alzheimer's disease. The importance of fostering mental activity to alleviate depressive symptoms cannot be overemphasized.

Groups that help older adults adapt to cultural changes in their lives alleviate much stress. The current changes in the delivery of health care, especially the movement toward managed health care, are markedly different from previous methods of third-party reimbursement for health care expenses. These changes make maneuvering through the health care system extremely difficult for older adults who grew up believing they always needed to respect the authority and judgment of physicians. They have become familiar with one physician upon whom they can rely and believe it is impolite or even disloyal to question his or her decisions. Being persistent, insisting upon having all their questions answered, and seeking another opinion are often unacceptable options.

Today's older adults require far different skills to navigate the health care system and to receive needed health care services. Adolph (1993) described her harrowing experience of dealing with her own physical limitations at age 77 in trying to obtain the medical help her dying husband needed from their health maintenance organization (HMO). She spoke of the depression, desperation, suicidal thoughts, and anger she felt at the physicians' indifference; lack of services granted by the HMO; and her terror at feeling so disempowered. Her story, eloquently told from her perspective as a former psychiatric social worker, is typical of many adults in today's society. Such experiences can be the source of many problems for elderly clients, and counselors must know how to identify and successfully solve them.

Group counseling designed to increase feelings of self-efficacy can help older adults learn and practice methods of self-care and cognitive self-talk; it also aids in the validation of each other's feelings to increase self-efficacy. Holahan and Holahan (1987) studied the relationship of self-efficacy and social support to adjustment in aging. A total of 52 elderly adults (65–75 years of age) who lived in a community participated in an initial structured interview and a follow-up interview 1 year later. The follow-up revealed that feelings of self-efficacy were related *inversely* to depression. Feelings of self-efficacy are central to initiating and maintaining behavior that enables older adults to obtain a sufficient level of social support. It follows that increased self-efficacy enables older adults to expand their support system.

Life Review:

Life review (Butler & Lewis, 1977) is a useful technique in elderly group work. As older adults relate life experiences, there is an opportunity to resolve old conflicts, express feelings surrounding painful past memories, and reconcile differences with family members. Life review can also renew a sense of strength, as clients are reminded of past accomplishments.

Reminiscence groups are also worthwhile in the treatment of depressive tendencies in older adults, both individually and in groups. Reminiscence training seems particularly useful as a deterrent to the learned helplessness (Seligman, 1975) or perceived loss of control over life situations often associated with depression and aging. Therapists can initiate reminiscence by asking group members to relate particularly stressful life events. The group leader leads the members to inquire about the strong feelings associated with these events and how they coped with them. Fry (1983) conducted research indicating that structured reminiscence was more beneficial for counselors than unguided or unstructured reminiscence. Fry trained counselors to pose specific questions about feelings, reactions, and the effects of remembered situations. Group members can be taught to recognize the skills and attributes used to cope with stressful events. Reframing the events is empowering, as group members realize they still possess the same qualities and characteristics that enabled them to overcome difficulties in their past.

Psychodrama:

Psychodrama is another constructive form for group therapy. Carman and Nordin (1984) reported the use of psychodrama, as developed by Moreno (1964), in the treatment of elderly adults in a nursing-home environment. The groups met for 1 hour and 15 minutes weekly for 14 months. During the warm-up phase, members shared experiences and selected a protagonist. Due to the physical limitations and frailties of the nursing-home residents, a vignette was used instead of action for the psychodrama phase. During the third phase, group members shared common emotional experiences and incidents. This action-oriented modality enabled group members to relive experiences, grieve losses, and express previously unexpressed feelings about events in their lives. Psychodrama also helped group members by fostering reminiscences and grief expression, reestablishing identities, as well as creating future projections. The authors also found that psychodrama simplified life reviews for participants.

Intergenerational:

Groups that center on intergenerational issues are quite beneficial. Intergenerational issues are frequent causes of concern for older adults and their children. Some of these difficulties can be attributed to cohort differences. In relationships with their children, many older persons have been socialized to believe that children should anticipate their parents' needs;

parents feel neglected when children do not respond to their needs. In reality, their children are most often unaware of either the needs or the disappointment. In families plagued by long-standing communication problems, elder adults often feel helpless to address the problems at hand. Although old hurts or grievances are causes of concern for older adults, they often do not know how to resolve such issues. Older parents may be aware that they are on poor terms with their adult children but fear making matters worse. They are afraid to talk directly with their children or even to try to make amends for past failures. Older adults become so fearful of inflaming their children that they refrain from talking to them with any depth of feeling. In such a situation, groups that help older adult parents deal with such issues and intergenerational groups that consist of older parents and adult children may be highly productive.

Intergenerational groups combining children and adolescents with older adults represent an effective variation of group counseling. Corey (1992) described an innovative group, designed by Nakkula, that combined older adults with adolescents. Through an eight-session program, Nakkula's aim was to assess individual changes in attitude based on the group experience. Posttesting revealed that the adolescents in the group had become much less biased toward older adults. At the same time, the older adults showed an increased sense of self-esteem. Also, the elders experienced much enjoyment from the opportunity to socialize with the adolescents, who, conversely, seemed to enjoy listening to the reminiscences of their elders.

In another intergenerational study, Generations Together collaborated with the Council Care Senior Adult Day Care (ADC) Centers in Pittsburgh and brought preschoolers, third-graders, and high-school students into 3 ADC centers once a week for 10-week cycles. Planned activities were conducted while the youngsters were present. The researchers found that preschool children had fewer negative stereotypes about the elderly, were more accepting and nonjudgmental, and enjoyed activities appropriate for the institutionalized older adults. In a music activity with young children, adult participants diagnosed with Alzheimer's disease displayed consistent positive behavior, responsiveness, and involvement that had not been displayed without the children. Staff members were amazed that formerly unresponsive patients smiled and reached out to the children. In even profoundly impaired patients, important behavioral changes were noted (Newman & Ward, 1993).

Bereavement:

Bereavement, or grief-resolution, groups provide an important tool in counseling older adults. Exploring the losses experienced and sharing feelings about these losses are the focus of the group. Grief over many types of losses can be addressed. The resulting grief from the loss of loved ones, careers, status, physical stamina, health, and so on can be shared and the process of grieving examined.

Levy, Derby, and Martinkowski (1993) investigated the contribution of membership in bereavement support groups to bereavement adaptation in a sample of 114 widows and 45 widowers. The mean age of the group members was 60.7 years. The group met for 18 months. The study found that the number of attended bereavement support group meetings accounted for a significant variance in the levels of anger and psychotropic medication used. As stated previously, loss (and the grief resulting from it) is one of the main themes influencing older adults.

Assertiveness Training:

Assertiveness training groups are another constructive technique for older adults. A potential trouble area, however, should be considered when counseling the elder married couple. Providing training to one member of a marriage without also providing some training to the spouse may evoke problems in the relationship. If one member suddenly begins acting assertively, a spouse who does not understand may be confused, threatened, and defensive.

Assertiveness training usually focuses first upon learning the assertive beliefs that facilitate assertiveness. This is followed by practice in acting assertively. We know that acting assertively increases personal competency and effectiveness; therefore, assertiveness training is especially helpful to older adults who have retired from major life work activities and may have few opportunities to practice assertive behavior. Many older adults have never acted assertively and may require this skill as they adjust to new living arrangements and taking care of themselves. Asking directly for what they want from family members, neighbors, salespeople, and others may be difficult. Many of today's cohorts of older adults were taught that it is impolite to be direct about one's feelings or preferences. Assertiveness training may help them understand the actions of their assertive children, grandchildren, and support personnel. As previously mentioned, older adults certainly need to act assertively in order to obtain needed health care.

Counseling and Exercise:

Another type of group for the treatment of depressive symptoms is the counseling and exercise group. Burlew, Jones, and Emerson (1991) organized a group counseling and exercise program. They posit that combining exercise with discussions of common problems associated with aging can alleviate depressive symptoms. It is widely recognized that physical exercise is a behavioral prescription for overcoming depression. Exercise seems to increase the release of endorphins in the brain and to generate a sense of personal power and increased well-being. Corey (1992) recommended the combination of group exercise and group counseling for older adults. Her program requires the exercise leader to take time during the exercise session to discuss whatever issues group members wish to discuss as a way of relieving depressive symptoms.

Counseling groups designed to help older adults adapt to diseases, such as diabetes mellitus, are especially useful. Containing the effects of disease requires considerable lifestyle adjustments. These adjustments are difficult to implement, and many confusing feelings may prevent compliance with stringent medical/behavioral management models.

Robinson (1993) conducted 12 structured group counseling sessions to help older adults with insulin-dependent diabetes lower their daily peak blood glucose levels. Five topics were introduced, and group discussions centered on each of these topics for two counseling sessions. Study results demonstrated the effectiveness of group counseling in helping older adults comply with their treatment plans and lower their blood glucose levels.

Groups that help older adults express negative feelings are theoretically beneficial in alleviating depression. For example, a link between anger and depression has long been postulated, although never proven. Accordingly, the relationship between anger expression and general health is a current area of study. Research seems to imply an association between negative emotions (such as anger and depression) and deleterious health outcomes. Although extremes in anger expression have been related to underlying health consequences, the suppression of emotional reactions is often linked to diseases involving the immune system, such as arthritis, diabetes, and hypertension (Linn, Linn, & Jensen, 1984). Williams and Williams (1993) have cited numerous studies asserting that emotions interact with interpersonal stress and personality variables and may become successful predictors of death due to cancer and cardiac disease. Groups that assist older adults to recognize and express strong emotions appropriately might relieve depressive symptoms.

Because our society devalues the status of older adults, their ability to influence their own lives may be diminished, including the ability to express emotions such as anger. In predisposed adults, repressed anger may be emotionally and physically debilitating. On the other hand, encouraging the proper expression of anger and giving older adults an increased measure of control in their lives may offset the toll taken by depression. Whether there is a link between anger and depression remains to be seen. There are indications that an age difference exists in expressing anger and hostility (Barefoot, Beckham, Haney, Siegler, & Lipkus, 1993), with older adults being less able to express anger. Findings also suggest that the negative effects of anger and depression are likely to have an impact upon the physical health and psychological well-being of older adults.

SUMMARY

It is important to remember that older adults are more heterogeneous than younger people. Their differences must be recognized in order for any mental health professional to offer effective help. Taking the time to become acquainted with older clients in order to understand what type of therapy might be most efficacious is imperative.

Group counseling appears to be an effective treatment modality for older adults with depressive symptoms. The group is an instrument for normalizing feelings and the aging process, providing needed support through the process of give and take. The diverse elderly population often has reduced opportunities for forming new relationships; because of fear of loss, many older adults are hesitant to make new friends.

The type of group counseling required depends upon the level of the client's impairment. Most older adults appear to benefit from some structure in the group counseling experience. Such structure can often take the form of an educational component. It takes time for group cohesiveness to reach a level at which that older adults feel safe enough to self-disclose, and the educational component allows time for inter-action prior to self-disclosure.

Depression is a debilitating condition for older adults in our society. Group counseling can be constructively used to com-bat depressive symptoms and prevent depression by increas-ing life satisfaction and self-efficacy. Forming new relation-ships with peers and becoming part of a support system are important components of counseling groups for older adults. Group counseling lessens the depressive side effects of coping with physical loss and the debilitation of chronic diseases. The support and encouragement of members of a counseling group strengthen the resolve of older adults to comply with the medical management of disease.

REFERENCES

Adolph, M. R. (1993). The myth of the golden years: One woman's perspective. *Women and Therapy, 14,* 55–66.

American Psychiatric Association. (1994). *Diagnostic and statistical manual of mental disorders* (4th ed.). Washington, DC: Author.

Aries, E. (1976). Interaction patterns and themes of male, female, and mixed groups. *Small Group Behavior, 7,* 7–18.

Association for Group Work. (1990). *Ethical guidelines for group counselors* (pp. 119–126). Alexandria, VA: American Counseling Association.

Barefoot, J. C., Beckham, J. C., Haney, T. L., Siegler, I. C., & Lipkus, I. M. (1993). Age differences in hostility among middle-aged and older adults. *Psychology and Aging, 8,* 3–9.

Belsky, J. K. (1984). *The psychology of aging: Theory, research, and practice.* Pacific Grove, CA: Brooks/Cole.

Brody, E. M. (1985). *Mental and physical health practices of older people.* New York: Springer.

Bruce, M. L., Leaf, P. J., Rozal, G. G., Florio, L., & Hoff, R. A. (1994). Psychiatric status and 9-year mortality data in the New Haven Epidemiologic Catchment Area study. *American Journal of Psychiatry, 151,* 716–721.

Burlew L. D., Jones, J., & Emerson, P. (1991). Exercise and the elderly: A group counseling approach. *The Journal for Specialists in Group Work, 16,* 152–158.

Butler, R., & Lewis, M. (1977). *Aging and mental health.* St. Louis, MO: CV Mosby.

Carman, M. B., & Nordin, S. R. (1984). Psychodrama: A therapeutic modality for the elderly in nursing homes. *Clinical Gerontologist, 3,* 15–24.

Corey, M. (1992). Groups for the elderly. In M. S. Corey & G. Corey (Eds.), *Groups: Process and practice* (pp. 399–430). Pacific Grove, CA: Brooks/Cole.

Fogel, B. S. (1991). Depression and aging. *Neuropsychiatry, Neuropsychology, and Behavioral Neurology, 4,* 24–35.

Fry, P. S. (1983). Structured and unstructured reminiscence training and depression among the elderly. *Gerontologist, 1,* 15–36.

Holahan, C. K., & Holahan, C. J. (1987). Self-efficacy, social support, and depression in aging: A longitudinal analysis. *Journal of Gerontology, 42,* 65–68.

Levy, L. H., Derby, J. F., & Martinkowski, K. S. (1993). Effects of membership in bereavement support groups on adaptation to conjugal bereavement. *American Journal of Community Psychology, 21,* 361–381.

Linn, M. W., Linn, B. S., & Jensen L. (1984). Stressful events, dysphoric mood, and immune responsiveness. *Psychological Reports, 54,* 219–222.

Miller, M. (1979). *Suicide after sixty: The final alternative.* New York: Springer.

Moreno, J. I. (1964). *Psychodrama.* New York: Beacon House.

Nelson, D. W. (1982). Alternative images of old age and the basis for policy. In B. L. Neugarten (Ed.), *Age or need?* (pp. 131-169). Beverly Hills, CA: Sage.

Newman, S., & Ward, C. (1993). An observational study of intergenerational activities and behavior change in dementing elders at adult day care centers. *International Journal of Aging and Human Development, 36*(4), 321–333.

Papolos, D. F., & Papolos, J. (1987). *Overcoming depression.* New York: Harper & Row.

Robinson, F. F. (1993). A training and support group for elderly diabetics: Description and evaluation. *The Journal for Specialists in Group Work, 18,* 127–136.

Schaie, K. W. (1965). A general model for the study of developmental problems. *Psychological Bulletin, 64,* 92–107.

Seligman, M. E. P. (1975). *Helplessness: On depression, development, and death.* San Francisco: W. H. Freeman.

Update on mood disorders — Part I. (1994). *Harvard Mental Health Letter, 11*(6), 1–4.

Williams R, & Williams V. (1993). *Anger kills.* New York: Random House.

Yalom, I. D. (1975). *The theory and practice of group psychotherapy.* New York: Basic Books.

Zarit, S. H. (1980). *Aging and mental disorders: Psychological approaches to assessment and treatment.* New York: Free Press.

6

The Risk of Misdiagnosing Physical Illness as Depression

Mark S. Gold, MD, FCP, FAPA

Dr. Gold is Professor, University of Florida Brain Institute, Departments of Neuroscience, Psychiatry, and Community Health & Family Medicine, Gainesville, FL.

KEY POINTS

- Many clients have a remarkably low response to the initial treatment of mental disorders. One of the major reasons for this is that they are misdiagnosed; they are actually suffering from a physical illness or from drug or alcohol abuse.

- Some common reasons that mental health professionals mistake physical illnesses for mental disorders are: their inability to deal with physical illness, lack of knowledge and continuing professional education, educational lag in training programs, and resistance to new information. Many disorders are on the borderline between mental health/ illness and internal medicine and neurology.

- Various physical illnesses and nutritional deficiencies that frequently appear to be mental disorders are reviewed.

- No matter how closely the first presentation of a mentally disabled client may conform to classic DSM-IV descriptive criteria, one cannot assume that the client is suffering from a psychiatric disorder.

- To reduce misdiagnosis and mistreatment of depression and other mental disorders, a complete physical, neurological, and endocrinological examination should be performed by a physician who is fluent in both psychiatry and internal medicine.

INTRODUCTION

One of the more recent discoveries of modern mental health care is that the majority of mental disorders show a remarkably low response to initial treatment (Shapiro & Keller, 1981). The rates of relapse of clients who are systematically followed for a period of a year or more is disconcerting (Hamilton, 1982; Shapiro & Keller, 1981). Such relapses are troublesome for both the client, who must ask for further treatment or switch therapists, and the professional, who must encounter a less cooperative client while trying to determine why the initial treatment failed.

One of the major reasons for treatment failures is that many clients are being treated for mental disorders when, in fact, they are suffering from physical illness, drug or alcohol abuse (Hall et al., 1978; Herridge, 1960; Koranyi, 1979), or dependence (Gold, 1992a, 1994; Gold & Gleaton, 1994; Gold & Miller, 1994; Miller & Gold, 1992). Psychiatric symptomatology can be, and frequently is, the first manifestation of a reversible physical illness.

Contrary to the beliefs of most medical professionals, clients whose mental symptoms mask physical illness are not rare. Although many psychotherapists contend that they have never seen cases of this sort, it has, in fact, been repeatedly documented by many different authors that physical illness needs to be vigorously excluded before a diagnosis of a mental illness can be made.

The *Diagnostic and Statistical Manual of Mental Disorders* (DSM-IV) (American Psychiatric Association, 1994) committee assumes that physical illnesses must be ruled out before proceeding through the decision tree (this is clear from looking at the DSM-IV differential diagnosis trees). If a physical illness is found, the diagnosis must then move into the section on organic mental disorders. Unfortunately, the most common misdiagnoses and the state-of-the-art workup for each are never addressed.

MISDIAGNOSIS: IS IT REALLY A PROBLEM?

Hall and associates (1978) studied 658 consecutive psychiatric outpatients; they found that 9.1% had medical disorders that produced mental, emotional, and behavioral symptoms. In an additional group of patients, medical disorders were mostly or partially causative. Forty-six percent of these patients could have been identified by their initial treating physicians, but they were not. In another study of outpatients, Koranyi (1979) excluded all patients who were immediately hospitalized as well as patients who failed to complete a comprehensive assessment. He started with an initial sample of 2670 patients; a final sample of 2090 patients who had been completely evaluated was examined. Forty-three percent of these patients were suffering from one or several major physical illnesses, 46% of which were undiagnosed at the time of referral; 7.74% of the total population had a physical illness that directly caused their psychiatric symptoms. Herridge (1960) studied 209 consecutive admissions to an inpatient unit and found that at least 5% had major physical illnesses that were causative of and presented as a psychiatric disorder.

Hall and colleagues (1981) conducted a prospective study of 100 admitted state hospital patients. Patients with known physical disorders along with sociopathic personality disorders and patients with significant histories of alcohol or drug abuse were omitted. An intensive search for causative physical illness revealed that 46% of the patients had a previously unrecognized and undiagnosed physical illness that was specifically related to their psychopathological symptoms and either caused these symptoms or substantially exacerbated them. Hall noted, ". . . 28 of 46 patients evidenced dramatic and rapid clearing of their mental/emotional symptoms when medical treatment for the underlying physical disorder was instituted. Eighteen patients were substantially improved immediately following appropriate medical treatments." The study of Hoffman (1982) yielded similar results: of 215 patients referred to a specialized medical psychiatric inpatient unit for further evaluation, the referring diagnosis was inaccurate in 41% of the cases, and 24% of cases were changed from physical to psychiatric or from psychiatric to physical illness.

Both medical and mental health professionals fail to diagnose physical illness. Koranyi (1979) reported that of all the sources referring clients to his outpatient clinic, medical personnel failed to find 32% of physical illness in referred clients, whereas psychiatrists missed 48% of physical illness in referred patients. Most striking was that 83%–83½% of all clients referred by social agencies or who were self-referred had undetected physical illness at the time they were seen in the outpatient department. Physicians are better than the patients themselves and other mental health workers in diagnosing physical illness, but their overall performance is poor by any standards (Dackis & Gold, 1984, 1986a; Extein & Gold, 1986; Gold, 1992b, 1993; Gross, Extein, & Gold, 1986; Miller, Mahler, & Gold, 1991).

These studies clearly show that physical illness is either a precipitant or associated condition that needs to be considered in any diagnostic formulation. More sophisticated and provocative testing techniques have been used successfully to help diagnose thyroid disease (Gold & Pearsall, 1983b) and identify low-dose drug and alcohol abuse among mental health clientele (Estroff & Gold, 1986b; Gold, 1989a, 1989b; Miller & Gold, 1991; Verebey, Gold, & Mule, 1986). These new tests will increase the percentage of detected medical illnesses (Extein & Gold, 1986; Gross, Extein, & Gold, 1986; Verebey, Martin, & Gold, 1987).

WHY MISDIAGNOSIS EXISTS

The factors leading to diagnostic errors are important and need to be scrutinized in detail. Many mental health professionals are unequipped to deal with physical illness in their clients. Klein and associates (1980) believed that errors in diagnosis "cannot be attributed to random sloppiness, bad faith, or lack of desire to help a patient to the utmost." They proposed a variety of reasons for why misdiagnosis occurs, including simple lack of knowledge, educational lag in training programs, lack of continuing professional education, and resistance to new information. This can lead to a selective rejection of certain facts of the case so that the client will more easily fit into the caregiver's specialty or orientation, which often results in a distortion and misperception of the client and his or her sometimes obvious physical illness. McIntyre and Romano (1977) found that less than 35% of practicing psychiatrists give their patients a physical examination. Thirty-two percent of psychiatrists admitted that they did not feel competent to perform even a rudimentary physical examination. However, these numbers may be much greater. Mental health professionals tend to consult either the client's family doctor, internist, pediatrician, or gynecologist for a medical clearance to rule out physical disorders.

The previously cited studies refer only to physical illnesses that presented as mental disorders and were, in whole or in part, causative of the mental symptoms. Physical illness can cause or worsen the symptoms of mental illness to a variable extent. Some disorders that present exclusively with symptoms of a mental disorder are wholly causative of the psychopathological symptomatology. These disorders, if they are treated properly and have not progressed to an irreversible stage, should result in a total clearing (a cure) of all such symptomatology without institution of nonphysical treatment. Other disorders exacerbate or, in part, cause the observed mental symptomatology, and, when treated, result in a significant but only partial clearing of the psychiatric symptoms. Still other illnesses are concomitant with and unrelated to the mental disorders, and, when treated, produce no effect on the mental symptoms. The group of psychopathological symptoms that develop in reaction to previously existing illness will be considered only in passing. Finally, some mental illnesses are often treated incorrectly as medical disorders by nonpsychiatric practitioners.

Many disorders are truly on the borderline between mental

health/illness and internal medicine and neurology. Most of these disorders are not detectable by physical examination or by "routine" laboratory screening alone. The correct diagnosis may not be made until the consulting physician is aware of the existence of these diseases and actively pursues the diagnosis through aggressive specialized testing. As many as 50 or 100 patients with apparently similar symptomatology may have to be tested to find 1 patient with a physical disorder. We believe this search is always worthwhile.

Misdiagnosis exists in the Prozac era because depression has been destigmatized and illicit drug addictions and alcoholism are seen as "abuses" and grounds for termination. Also, pharmacological treatment advances have been rapid in affective, panic, obsessive compulsive disorder (OCD), and other psychiatric disorders, yet the current treatment of choice for alcoholics is evaluation, detoxification, Alcoholics Anonymous (AA), and abstinence. Many alcoholics and drug abusers are treated for "depression" with antidepressants or other agents out of treatment bias.

SPECIFICITY OF PRESENTING PSYCHOPATHOLOGICAL SYMPTOMS

From the previously cited studies, and many others, it becomes clear that no matter how closely the first presentation of a mentally disabled client may conform to classic DSM-IV descriptive criteria, one cannot assume that the client is suffering from a psychiatric disorder.

This nonspecificity of medical disease causing specific syndromes is particularly true for depressive disorders. The differential diagnosis of depression is long and involved. Giannini, Black, and Goettsche (1978) listed 91 possible disorders that can present as depression. Hall (1980) listed 24 medical illnesses that frequently induce depression and 77 medical conditions that can present as depression.

To summarize thus far, many clients who present with mental/emotional symptomatology actually have medical illnesses. The psychiatric symptoms are merely the first and most obvious manifestation of the physical illness. No psychopathological sign or symptom is pathognomonic of a mental disorder to the extent that it cannot be caused by a physical disorder. Many nonpsychiatric physicians and mental health professionals, including psychiatrists, are either unaware of these facts or choose to ignore them. A diagnosis of mental disorder is only made by exhaustive evaluation. Simply meeting descriptive criteria does not confirm such a diagnosis at any time. Most clients who present with mental/emotional symptoms are not given a thorough physical examination and medical workup to detect possible medical causes of the psychiatric symptoms, which would then be reversed by treating the primary disease.

MEDICAL ILLNESSES THAT MAY PRESENT AS MENTAL DISORDERS

The following section will review various medical disorders that can present psychopathologically and mimic any depressive illness.

The Carcinoid Syndrome:

Carcinoid tumor may be confused with major depression, hypomania, major depression with psychosis, or anxiety. It may not always be accompanied by spontaneous flushing of the upper body precipitated by consuming certain foods or alcohol, epinephrine administration, excitement, or exertion. An attack may be accompanied by abdominal pain and diarrhea. The syndrome accompanies a variety of tumors that can occur in the gastrointestinal tract and lungs and that secrete various biologically active substances, including dopamine, histamine, corticotropin (ACTH), and serotonin. Serotonin-secreting tumors are most common.

If this disorder is included in the differential diagnosis, the diagnosis may be confirmed by an increased urinary excretion of 5-hydroxyindoleacetic acid (5-HIAA), which normally does not exceed 9 mg daily.

Cancer:

Many patients with malignant tumors may present to the mental health professional with depressive symptomatology, often meeting DSM-IV criteria months or even years earlier than physical symptoms or signs.

Of all the malignant tumors that present psychopathologically, pancreatic carcinoma is the most notorious (Jefferson & Marshall, 1981). The first signs of the tumor are often severe depression with crying spells, insomnia unresponsive to sleeping medication, and anxiety associated with the fear that the patient has a very serious illness.

Central nervous system (CNS) tumors present with mental/emotional symptomatology, especially if they occur in the temporal and frontal regions. The most common symptom is a change in personality. Left-sided tumors present more frequently as irritability or depression, whereas tumors of the parietal and occipital lobes tend to be relatively silent. Limbic system tumors can present as depression, delusions, assaultive behavior, and confusional states. Human immunodeficiency virus (HIV) infection in the central nervous system and right-sided cerebrovascular accidents (CVAs) can mimic depression, anxiety, and panic attacks. A high index of suspicion is indicated when the client presents in an atypical fashion with a personality change, depression with a weight loss greater than 20 pounds, or is unresponsive to a first trial of standard mental health care.

Diabetes Mellitus:

In a study by Hall and colleagues (1981), certain clients with diabetes mellitus presented psychiatrically and met the diagnostic criteria for major depression, and for other disorders as well. Diabetes may present as depression, sexual dysfunction, and/or marital problems (Gold, 1995). The diagnosis is made by demonstrating an elevated fasting blood sugar or an abnormal response to a glucose load at 1 and 2 hours.

Illicit Drugs:

Drug (Gold, 1995) and alcohol abuse (Dackis and Gold, 1986b) and withdrawal may imitate depressive illnesses. Furthermore, hospitalized psychiatric patients sometimes abuse drugs in the hospital, resulting in confusing changes in function and severe exacerbations of their illnesses (Miller, Hoffman, & Gold, 1994). The only way to make the drug abuse diagnosis is to be constantly aware of the frequency of drug and alcohol problems. Simply questioning the client without formal testing is both naïve and dangerous. Drug intoxication, drug withdrawal, and the sequelae of drug abuse should be actively eliminated from consideration (Gold, Pottash, & Extein, 1982). Such clients commonly present with symptoms of depression, and they may meet the DSM-IV criteria for major depression. Drug abuse can, however, resemble any known condition from psychosis to mild anxiety states and must be considered in all psychiatric disorders no matter how classic the presentation. Asking the client about the existence and extent of drug use is essential; however, anecdote should never be confused with fact. Drug use, drug intoxication, and drug withdrawal diagnosis should be confirmed whenever possible by blood or urine testing.

Nicotine and alcohol abuse, dependence, and involvement are also common causes of misdiagnosis and failure to respond to treatment. Nicotine dependence is decreasing in response to widespread public education and the availability of successful smoking cessation programs. This decrease has been most pronounced among the most well-educated citizens in the United States. When a cigarette-smoking nurse, therapist, or physician is identified and detoxified (or fail in detoxification), underlying depression may be found to be the cause. Patients with depression who smoke cigarettes, may be found to be nonresponders because their nicotine dependence has not been treated. Cigarette smoking can interfere not only with

medication response by altering the metabolism of the antidepressant; it can make treatment difficult in many cases.

Alcoholic patients generally meet DSM-IV criteria for major
depressive disorder. If a person does not know that he or she
is an alcoholic, treatment will fail. Alcoholics often have depressed moods and disturbed sleep and appetite — symptoms
commonly associated with naturally occurring depression.

Many frequent users of marijuana experience anxiety and
complain of memory loss and affective changes. This is becoming more true as the THC (tetrahydrocannabinol) level has
increased in the typical marijuana cigarette. MDMA, or ectasy,
the use of which is widespread at "raves," or all-night dance
parties packed with participants fueled on various hallucinogenic drugs (Gold, in press), is associated with panic and
anxiety, which can persist long after MDMA use is discontinued. Similarly, the resurgence in LSD (lysergic acid) use has
made the diagnosis of psychosis all the more difficult (Gold, in
press).

Prescription Drugs:

Psychopathological symptoms occur in at least 2.7% of
patients taking prescription medication on a regular basis,
according to the Boston Collaborative Drug Surveillance Study
of 9000 patients (Extein & Gold, 1986).

**Hyperadrenalism (Cushing's Syndrome) and
Hypoadrenalism (Addison's Disease):**

Cushing's syndrome may present as an affective illness
with or without psychosis, euphoria, or anxiety. In one study
using structured interviews and RDC criteria, depression was
present in 83% of patients with endogenous Cushing's syndrome who met RDC criteria for either mania or hypomania
prior to the depression (Gold, 1995).

Hypoadrenalism commonly presents as depression or organic brain syndrome. The diagnosis is usually made on the
basis of low diurnal serum cortisol and low 24-hour urine

cortisol excretion. Hypoadrenalism is easily treated with steroid replacement therapy.

Hypoglycemia:

Many people diagnose themselves as hypoglycemic in order to explain their depressive symptomatology. There is little proof that all such clients have symptomatic hypoglycemia. However, there are several conditions that can cause symptomatic hypoglycemia. The most prominent are insulinoma and the exogenous administration of insulin. Insulinoma is probably the most frequent cause of symptomatic hypoglycemia and may produce bizarre behavior that can be indistinguishable from schizophrenia, depression, dementia, or anxiety attacks.

Hyperparathyroidism and Hypoparathyroidism:

The mental/emotional disturbances seen in hyperparathyroidism are directly related to serum calcium levels. Serum calcium levels of 12 to 16 mg/100 mL are associated with psychopathological changes (Extein & Gold, 1986; Gross, Estein, & Gold, 1986). Hypoparathyroidism with resultant low serum calcium levels most commonly presents as an organic brain syndrome, but it may appear to be delirium tremens or depression with psychosis. Diagnosis of both hyperparathyroidism and hypoparathyroidism is first suspected upon seeing an abnormal serum calcium level on routine blood screening or from a history of thyroid or parathyroid disorders in the family and/or previous thyroid or parathyroid surgery.

Hyperthyroidism and Hypothyroidism:

Hyperthyroidism may resemble panic disorder, anxiety, neurosis, or mania. People fail to realize that hyperthyroidism frequently presents as depression. The diagnosis of hyperthyroidism is made by the classical symptoms of hyperthyroidism, along with elevated T_3 and T_4, a depressed level of thyroid-stimulating hormone (TSH), and a low TSH response to thytroprin-releasing hormone (TRH) administration.

Hypothyroidism has been classically associated with psychosis in the form of "myxedema madness." It is also associated with depression and organic brain syndromes. Gold and Pearsall (1983b) demonstrated that there is a subtle form of hypothyroidism, "subclinical hypothyroidism," in which all the thyroid function tests, including T_3, T_4, and T_3 uptake, and TSH are normal in the presence of exaggerated TSH response to the administration of intravenous TRH. Patients with an augmented TSH and titers of thyroid autoantibodies have successfully been treated with thyroid hormone alone. Furthermore, symptomless autoimmune thyroiditis (SAT), a discrete syndrome, exists in 7%-15% of inpatients and outpatients who meet DSM-IV criteria for major depression (Gold, 1995). Thyroid abnormalities and subclinical hypothyroidism have been identified as a cause of rapid cycling in bipolar disease (Extein & Gold, 1988; Goodnick, Estein, & Gold, 1988; Gross, Extein, & Gold, 1986; Gold, 1994; Miller & Gold, 1994).

Metal Poisonings:

Heavy metal poisoning can occur with environmental exposure to or ingestion of a wide variety of metals, including magnesium, copper, zinc, manganese, lead, mercury, thallium, bismuth, aluminum, arsenic, and bromides. Most consistently, these metals produce an organic brain syndrome but can also mimic major depression.

Unless they are actively looked for with heavy metal screens by atomic absorption or plasma emission spectroscopy of urine and blood, these metals will not be found and properly treated. If such conditions are detected and treated early enough, the mental and emotional symptoms are, for the most part, reversible.

Huntington's Disease:

A high incidence of symptoms resembling both mania and

depression is common in patients with Huntington's disease. This was noted even in Huntington's original article of 1872: "The tendency to insanity and sometimes that form of insanity which leads to suicide is marked." Like other diseases from hypothyroidism to folate or B_{12} deficiency, psychiatric manifestations of this disease can occur well before any of the choreiform movements or any of the signs of dementia.

Infectious Mononucleosis:

Infectious mononucleosis may be followed by a syndrome that is identical to a major depressive episode. The diagnosis of infectious mononucleosis is made by a positive heterophile or mono spot test. A single negative test never excludes the diagnosis.

Infectious Hepatitis:

Mental and emotional symptoms before, during, or after infectious hepatitis of any type, A, B, or non-A non-B, can range from mild lethargy to major depression. There are even some reports of suicide and acute delusional mania following hepatitis.

Multiple Sclerosis:

Multiple sclerosis (MS) is a demyelinating neurologic disease characterized by lesions that are separated in space and time within the central nervous system. MS has been associated with a wide variety of psychopathological symptomatology, including mania and depression.

Panhypopituitarism:

Psychiatric presentations are common in pituitary failure and usually present with depression and/or lack of libido.

Postconcussion Syndrome:

The postconcussion syndrome occurs as the aftereffects of brain damage from severe head injury. It may present as anxiety, depression, excess anger, loss of emotional control, mood swings from euphoria to depression, and social disinhibition. Lesions of the left hemisphere, especially the left temporal lobe, tend to produce more intellectual deficits, whereas affective and behavioral symptoms are more frequently observed in right-hemisphere damage.

Syphilis (General Paresis):

At one time, syphilis accounted for 10%–20% of all admissions to state hospitals for the insane. This makes penicillin one of the most important psychiatric treatments of all time (Estroff & Gold, 1986a; Extein & Gold, 1987).

Systemic Lupus Erythematosus:

Systemic lupus erythematosus is a relatively uncommon disease that occurs in 2–3 per 100,000 population, with a 9:1 ratio favoring females (Gross, Extein, & Gold, 1986). It can present any time between ages 10 and 70 and may be accompanied by a wide variety of psychiatric symptoms, including mania, depression, schizophreniform or schizophrenic psychosis, and organic brain syndrome; it may even be labelled as a conversion disorder (Gross, Extein, & Gold, 1986). Systemic lupus erythematosus is too often overlooked in young women presenting with emotional symptoms and complaining of arthralgias, despite the fact that arthralgias are the most common first presentation of this disorder.

Vitamin Deficiencies:

Among the better known vitamin deficiencies associated with mental and emotional symptoms are folate (Hall et al., 1981; Jefferson & Marshall, 1981), vitamin B_{12} deficiency

(Jefferson & Marshall, 1981), and niacin (nicotine acid). Folic-acid deficiency presents with depression, fatigue, and lassitude. Marked deficiency can present with burning feet, restless leg syndrome, and/or a depression that is unresponsive to antidepressant therapy. Coppen and Abou-Saleh (1982) found a higher rate of affective morbidity in patients with low folate levels than patients with normal folate levels in patients treated in a lithium clinic. Hall and colleagues (1981), in a prospective study of hospitalized state psychiatric patients, found three cases of folate deficiency, two of which presented as RDC schizophrenia and one as RDC schizoaffective disorder. Normal CBC (complete blood cell count) folate deficiency occurs frequently and is often misdiagnosed and mistreated.

A deficiency of vitamin B_{12} may also present psychopathologically in the absence of any signs of anemia or bone marrow changes. It may present neurologically as a peripheral neuropathy or myelopathy (subacute combined degeneration). It has been known to present with a wide spectrum of mental and emotional disorders, including apathy, irritability, depression, dementia, confusional states, paranoid states, and schizophreniform psychosis (Jefferson & Marshall, 1981).

Patients who develop a zinc deficiency may become depressed, complain of lost interest in food, and show weight loss.

THE RELATIVE FREQUENCY OF OCCURRENCE OF NONPSYCHIATRIC ILLNESS PRESENTING AS PSYCHOPATHOLOGICAL SYMPTOMS

Symptoms of depression caused by the use of drugs, alcohol, and other substances appear to be the most common cause of psychiatric misdiagnosis and mistreatment. As a general category, endocrine disorders present most frequently in association with depressive symptoms. Provocative testing will make that point even more evident in the future. The second most commonly involved organ system is the central nervous system. Toxic and withdrawal disorders were found third most commonly. Nutritional disorders and infectious diseases are the fourth most common. Cancer and metabolic disorders, such as Wilson's disease, acute intermittent porphyria, G6 PDase deficiency, and polycystic ovaries, exist but are rare unless the client has an unusual presentation, recent treatment failure, atypical features, or 20 pounds or more weight loss.

SUMMARY

To reduce misdiagnosis and mistreatment of depression and other mental disorders, a complete physical, neurological, and endocrinological examination should be performed by a physician who is fluent in both psychiatry and internal medicine. This examination should be directed toward finding possible addictive, physical, or other illnesses that might cause or exacerbate mental and emotional symptoms (Gold, 1992a, 1994; Gold & Gleaton, 1994; Gold & Miller, 1994; Miller & Gold, 1992).

The laboratory is becoming an important component of any evaluation (Gold, 1995), but it does not replace the physician. Lab tests are ordered to correspond to and confirm the major issues in the differential diagnosis, and they may reveal unsuspected diagnostic clues.

A common model of care is to establish a clinical diagnosis and then treat the patient. For example, patients who meet DSM-IV criteria for major depressive episode may be treated with the selective serotonin reuptake inhibitors (SSRIs) by primary care and other physicians. Failure to respond to the appropriate psychopharmacological treatment of the diagnosis, therefore, is a very important indicator; it suggests that the diagnosis is incorrect and that the patient is in a high-risk group for underlying and undiagnosed exacerbating or precipitated illness.

The mental health practice is likely to change radically in the future. We hope that the information contained in this chapter and reported elsewhere in greater detail (Gold, Lydiard, & Carman, 1984) will help present and future mental health professionals make this change to more easily.

REFERENCES

American Psychiatric Association. (1994). *Diagnostic and statistical manual of mental disorders* (4th ed.). Washington, DC: Author.

Coppen, A., & Abou-Saleh, M. T. (1982). Plasma folate and affective morbidity during long-term lithium therapy. *British Journal of Psychiatry, 141,* 87-89.

Dackis, C. A., & Gold, M. S. (1984). Depression in opiate addicts. In S. M. Mirin (Ed.), *Substance abuse and psychopathology* (pp. 20-39). Washington: American Psychiatric Press, Inc.

Dackis, C. A., & Gold, M. S. (1986a). The self-medication hypothesis of addictive disorders: Focus on heroin and cocaine dependence. [Letters to the editor.] *American Journal of Psychiatry, 143*(10), 1309.

Dackis, C. A., & Gold, M. S. (1986b). Evaluating depression in alcoholics. *Psychiatry Research, 17,* 105-109.

Estroff, T. W., & Gold, M. S. (1986a). Medication-induced and toxin-induced psychiatric disorder. In I. Extein & M. S. Gold (Eds.), *Medical mimics of psychiatric disorders* (chap. 7, pp. 163-198). Washington, DC: American Psychiatric Press.

Estroff, T. W., & Gold, M. S. (1986b). Psychiatric presentations of marijuana abuse. *Psychiatric Annals, 16*(4), 221-224.

Extein, I., & Gold. M. S. (Eds.) (1986). *Medical mimics of psychiatric disorders.* Washington, DC: APA Press.

Extein, I., & Gold. M. S. (1987, April). *Endocrinological diseases mimicking affective disorders.* Paper presented at the International Conference on New Directions in Affective Disorders, Jerusalem, Israel.

Extein, I., & Gold. M. S. (1988). Thyroid hormone potentiation of tricyclics. *Psychosomatics, 29*(2), 167-174.

Giannini, A. J., Black H. R., & Goettsche, R. L. (1978). *Psychiatric, psychogenic, and somatopsychic disorders handbook.* New York: Medical Examination Publishing Co.

Gold, M. S. (1989a). *Drugs of abuse: A comprehensive series for clinicians. Vol. I. Marijuana.* New York & London: Plenum.

Gold, M. S. (1989b). *The good news about panic, anxiety, and phobias.* New York: Villard & Bantam Books.

Gold, M. S. (1992a). Seeking drugs/alcohol and avoiding withdrawal: The neuroanatomy of drive states and withdrawal. *Psychiatric Annals, 22,* 430-435.

Gold, M. S. (1992b). Cocaine (and crack). In J. Lowinson, P. Ruiz, & R. Millman (Eds.), *Clinical aspects in substance abuse: A comprehensive textbook.* (2nd ed., pp. 205-221). Baltimore: Williams & Wilkins.

Gold, M. S. (1993). Distinguishing psychiatric syndromes in alcoholism. In M. Aronson, *Alcoholism: Recognition of the disease and considerations for patient care* (pp. 24-27). Rancho Mirage, CA: Betty Ford Center.

Gold, M. S. (1994). The epidemiology, attitudes, and pharmacology of LSD use in the 1990s. *Psyciatric Annals, 24*(3), 124-126.

Gold, M. S. (1995). *The good news about depression.* New York: Bantam Books.

Gold, M. S. (in press). Trends in hallucinogenic drug use: LSD, 'Ecstasy,' and the rave phenomenon. In *The Hatherleigh Guide to Substance Abuse I.* New York: Hatherleigh Press.

Gold, M. S., & Gleaton, T. J. (1994). Marked increases in USA marijuana and LSD: Results of an annual junior and senior high school survey. *Biological Psychiatry, 35*(9), 694.

Gold, M. S., & Herridge, P. (1988). The risk of misdiagnosing physical illness as depression. In F. Flach (Ed.), *Affective disorders* (chap. 7, pp. 64-76). New York: W. W. Norton & Co.

Gold, M. S., Lydiard, R. B., & Carman, J. S. (Eds.). (1984). *Advances in psychopharmacology: Predicting and improving treatment response.* Boca Raton, FL: CRC Press.

Gold, M. S., & Miller, N. S. (1994). The biology of addictive and psychiatric disorders. In N. S. Miller (Ed.), *Treating coexisting psychiatric and addictive disorders* (pp. 35-52). Center City, MN: Hazelden.

Gold, M. S. & Pearsall, H. R. (1983a). Depression and hypothyroidism. *JAMA, 250*(18), 2470-2471.

Gold, M. S., & Pearsall, H. R. (1983b). Hypothyroidism—Or is it depression? *Psychosomatics, 24,* 646-654.

Gold, M. S., Pottash, A. C., & Extein, I. (1982). The psychiatric laboratory. In J. G. Bernstein (Ed.), *Clinical psychopharmacology* (pp. 29-58). Boston: John Wright PSG.

Goodnick, P. J., Extein, I., & Gold, M. S. (1988, March). Subclinical moods in substance abuse. *American Psychopathological Association poster session.* New York: American Psychopathological Association.

Gross, D. A., Extein, I., & Gold, M. S. (1986). The psychiatrist as physician. In I. Extein & M. S. Gold (Eds.), *Medical mimics of psychiatric disorders* (pp. 1-12). Washington, DC: American Psychiatric Association.

Hall, R. C. W., et al. (1978). Physical illness presenting as psychiatric disease. *Archives of General Psychiatry, 35,* 1315-1320.

Hall, R. C. W. (1980). *Psychiatric presentations of medical illness.* New York: Spectrum.

Hall, R. C. W., et al. (1981). Unrecognized physical illness prompting psychiatric admission: A prospective study. *American Journal of Psychiatry, 138,* 629-635.

Hamilton, M. (1982). The effect of treatment on the melancholias (depressions). *British Journal of Psychiatry, 140,* 223-230.

Herridge, C. F. (1960). Physical disorders in psychiatric illness: A study of 209 consecutive admissions. *Lancet, 2,* 949-951.

Hoffman, R. S. (1982). Diagnostic errors in the evaluation of behavioral disorders. *Journal of the American Medical Association, 248,* 964-967.

Jefferson, J. W., & Marshall, J. R. (1981). *Neuropsychiatric features of medical disorders.* New York: Plenum.

Koranyi, E. K. (1979). Morbidity and rate of undiagnosed physical illness in a psychiatric clinic population. *Archives of General Psychiatry, 36,* 414-449.

Klein, D. F., Gittelman, R., Quitkin, F., & Rifkin, A. (1980). *Diagnosis and drug treatment of psychiatric disorders: Adults and children.* Baltimore: Williams & Wilkins.

McIntyre, J. W., & Romano, J. (1977). Is there a stethoscope in the house (and is it used)? *Archives of General Psychiatry, 34*, 1147-1151.

Miller, N. S., & Gold, M. S. (1991). *Drugs of abuse: A comprehensive series for clinicians. Vol. II. Alcohol.* New York & London: Plenum.

Miller, N. S., & Gold, M. S. (1992). The psychiatrist's role in integrating pharmacological and nonpharmacological treatments for addictive disorders. *Psychiatric Annals, 22*(8), 436-440.

Miller, N. S., & Gold, M. S. (1994). LSD and ecstacy: Pharmacology, phenomenology, and treatment. *Psychiatric Annals, 24*(3), 131-133.

Miller, N. S., Hoffmann, N. G., & Gold, M. S. (1994). Comorbid depression, drug dependence, and alcoholism. *Society for Neuroscience Abstract, 20*, 1609.

Miller, N. S., Mahler, J. C., & Gold, M. S. (1991). Suicide risk associated with drug and alcohol dependence. *Journal of Addictive Diseases, 10*(3), 49-61.

Shapiro, R. W., & Keller, M. B. (1981). Initial 6-month follow-up of patients with major depressive disorder. *Journal of Affective Disorders, 3*, 205-220.

Verebey, K., Gold, M. S., & Mule, S. J. (1986). Laboratory testing in the diagnosis of marijuana intoxication and withdrawal. *Psychiatric Annals, 16*(4), 235-241.

Verebey, K., Martin, D., & Gold, M. S. (1987). Interpretation of drug abuse testing: Strengths and limitations of current methodology. *Psychiatric Medicine, 3*(3), 287-297.

7

Principles in Psychotherapy for Depression

Louis Jolyon West, MD

Dr. West is Professor of Psychiatry, UCLA School of Medicine, Los Angeles, CA.

KEY POINTS

- *Integrative psychotherapy* is based on the twin concepts that every depressed client can benefit from treatment and psychotherapy should play a part in every case, regardless of other modalities being employed.

- The goal of integrative psychotherapy is to promote the client's integrity in three senses (functional wholeness, existential continuity, and adaptational relevance) through the coordinated use of methods that are scientifically derived, client centered, and professionally committed.

- The four principal components in the general strategy of integrative psychotherapy of depres-

sion are rapport, reassurance, revelation, and reorganization.

- Every symptom of depressive illness can be manifested in certain cases of bereavement. Treatment should be based on the principles of integrative psychotherapy with special considerations and areas of emphasis.

- The integrative psychotherapy for depression should be focused and time limited; however, it should not be terminated abruptly. The client's own perception of his or her need for continued contact should be used as a guide when discussing cessation of treatment.

Portions of this chapter are adapted from: West, L. J. (1975). Integrative psychotherapy of depressive illness. In F. F. Flach & S. C. Draghi (Eds.), The nature and treatment of depression (pp. 161-181). New York: John Wiley & Sons. Adapted with permission from F. F. Flach.

INTRODUCTION

Depression is a symptom rather than a disease, even though some diseases may be named after it. The indications and contraindications for treating depression should be based on an understanding of the cause-and-effect relationships underlying the development of the condition. This holds true even when the treatment itself is empirical — as in the use of techniques such as interpersonal psychotherapy, behavior therapy, or pharmacotherapy for the relief of symptoms — and when symptomatic relief is the client's only stated desire.

There are dozens of contemporary psychotherapies defined by different names; they all have characteristics in common. Sometimes the distinctions between them are minor, to the point of apparent irrelevance; sometimes the differences are profound. Virtually every type of psychotherapy has been used for the treatment of depression. Therefore, a brief look at the classification of psychotherapies is appropriate.

At least seven criteria for classifying psychotherapies can be identified:

1. Psychotherapies may be classified according to the *conceptual orientation* of the therapist. Such conceptualizations usually derive from the teachings of their originators (e.g., Freudian, Jungian, Kleinian, and Myerian). Psychoanalysis and the various psychoanalytically oriented modifications of it (e.g., *dynamic* psychotherapies), as well as various other interpersonal therapies, such as the techniques described by Klerman, Weissman, Rounsaville, and Chevron (1984), are excellent examples of conceptual classification.

2. Psychotherapies may also be named in accordance with *phenomenologic and quantitative signs and symptoms* and behavioral manifestations of psychopathology, together with the direct process of chang-

ing them (e.g., behavior therapies and behavior modification techniques).

3. A third approach to the classification of psychotherapies emphasizes the *structural circumstances of treatment,* especially (but not necessarily) if it is other than one-to-one. Thus, we find references to group therapy, family therapy, marital therapy, and so forth.

4. Another method of classifying psychotherapies places emphasis on *the employment of a particular treatment technique,* such as hypnotherapy, psychodrama, and narcosynthesis.

5. A fifth classification emphasizes *crucial events or experiences* that are expected or produced in the course of treatment. Catharsis and gestalt therapy are examples.

6. A sixth approach stresses the *circumstances or constraints* under which treatment takes place: emergency psychotherapy, brief psychotherapy, crisis intervention, and the like.

7. A seventh way of classifying psychotherapies is based on *the goals of treatment;* for instance, supportive therapy, insight therapy, and reality therapy.

SELECTION OF CASES

Advocates of these psychotherapies vary in their willingness to limit the use of their particular method according to the nature of the illness. For example, nonprofessional psychotherapists are notoriously global in their approach and believe that their particular method would benefit anyone, regardless of his or her condition. On the other hand, orthodox psychoanalysts are likely to look for a number of characteristics in the client that suggest suitability for treatment by their method, such as a diagnosis of neurotic depressive reaction as opposed to manic-depressive disorder.

West (1975) described an approach to psychotherapy called *integrative psychotherapy* that is applicable in all — or nearly all — cases of depression. It is an approach based on the twin concepts that every depressed client can benefit from treatment, and that a well-trained general psychotherapist can treat any depressed client if he or she must, at least to the point that collaboration with a specialist (e.g., in psychopharmacology or electroconvulsive therapy [ECT]) is indicated.

INTEGRATIVE PSYCHOTHERAPY

Integrative psychotherapy might be classified under more than one of the seven groups listed herein. The approach is integrative in two ways: the *goals* of treatment and the *process* of treatment.

The *goal* of integrative psychotherapy is to promote the client's integrity in three senses: functional wholeness, existential continuity, and adaptational relevance. *Functional wholeness* implies a healing process, the restoration and promotion of healthy personality function in mood, thought, and behavior. *Existential continuity* is an educational, maturational, growth-provoking process that restores and promotes integration of the client's personal lessons of the past for comprehension of the present and future. *Adaptational relevance* means a balanced, harmonious relationship with the physical, social, and moral environment. In this sense, integrative psychotherapy is a philosophically and ethically enriching process that restores and promotes humane sensibilities.

The *process* of integrative psychotherapy connotes the coordinated use of methods that are scientifically derived, client centered, and professionally committed. *Scientifically derived* therapy is applied knowledge that uses information from the basic biomedical and psychosocial sciences and focuses that knowledge upon specific human problems. The process is *client centered* because it integrates various appropriate treatment techniques, singly or in combination, and constantly revalidates or modifies them according to their actual effectiveness in each individual case. Similar to the interpersonal psychotherapy of Klerman and colleagues (1984), it emphasizes current relationships, even while considering the roles of genetic, metabolic, developmental, and characterologic factors in predisposition and development. *Professional commitment* implies the ethical integrity of the therapist who incorporates various requirements for ethical safeguards during treatment, interpersonal responsibilities in the therapist-client relationship, and the simultaneous social responsibilities of a licensed professional.

The integrative psychotherapy for depression must deliberately integrate various data, methodologies, techniques, and values into a consistent whole. The primary thrust of treatment is directed toward depression, whether it be the primary problem or a symptom of another psychopathologic disorder. Because much treatment of depressive illness is still empirical and symptomatic, formulating general psychotherapeutic guidelines for all clients with depressive symptomatology is recommended.

GENERAL ELEMENTS IN PSYCHOTHERAPY FOR DEPRESSION

There are four "R's" in the general strategy of integrative psychotherapy for depression: rapport, reassurance, revelation, and reorganization.

Rapport:

Because depression poses unusual problems in the therapist-client relationship, the therapist must make an exceptional effort to establish rapport with his or her depressed client. The client may feel unworthy or hopeless, or otherwise unable to become trusting or close. The element of anxiety that may foster relief through an early positive transference in some neurotic disorders is much less likely to produce such a result when depression is present to a significant degree. In developing good rapport, it is important to use every possible point of contact with the depressed client. This may require considerable study of his or her family, business, hobbies, and personal history.

Reassurance:

The depressed client has a genuine need for reassurance, even if he or she seems unable to take much comfort from it. The therapist should be prepared to express reassurance repeatedly in a calm, nonirritated fashion. To be most effective, reassurance should be more than verbal. Many routine activities, including occupational and recreational therapies for the hospitalized depressed client, can exert a valuable reassuring effect. Physical exercise has a positive benefit, not only because of salubrious psychophysiologic effects, but also because it exerts a constant reassurance to the client that he or she will once again be capable of vigorous and constructive action. Numerous other reassuring maneuvers will present themselves in each individual case.

Revelation:

The process of self-discovery is intrinsic to all dynamic psychotherapies. The mental content of the depressed client frequently includes ruminations over putative discoveries that are ego-dystonic. The therapist must deal with such depressive revelations, or pseudorevelations, and incorporate them into an overall strategy of improved self-understanding for the client. This may range from increased, but fairly limited, awareness of the self in some cases to profound emotional insight in others.

Reorganization:

Reorganization refers to both the personality of the client and his or her lifestyle. It is often necessary to spend considerable time assembling, synthesizing, and integrating the total experience of the client after the depressed mood has lifted, but before he or she is ready to resume full, normal living. An important component of this will often prove to be the formulating of specific plans for a healthier organization of the client's post-illness life, taking into account the risk of future depressions and reviewing preventative measures, early warning signs, and procedures for instituting early intervention, if needed, in the event of a recurrence.

PSYCHOTHERAPY AND MEDICATION

Recent studies have compared various forms of psychotherapy with pharmacotherapy, either alone or in combination, and have found that all forms of therapy are effective in treating depression (Robinson, Berman, & Neimeyer, 1990; Starvynski & Greenberg, 1992). However, characteristics of individual clients may make one form more effective than another (Sotsky et al., 1991). Drugs act more quickly and may be more specific in treating the somatic and vegetative symptoms of depression, whereas psychotherapies are more likely to effect change in the psychosocial and cognitive aspects. Because the overall strategy of integrative psychotherapy is governed by each client's needs, resources, and potentialities, antidepressant medication can often play an important adjunctive role in the treatment of the depressed client. However, psychotherapy should be a significant part of every depressed client's treatment, even if it is employed mainly during follow-up visits in cases where physiologic or pharmacologic interventions were apparently primary.

MANAGING SUICIDAL RISK

To a greater or lesser degree, every depressed client poses some risk of self-destruction. This issue must be made explicit from the very beginning of the therapeutic relationship. It should be discussed often, appropriately, and in detail. A common misconception about suicide holds that persons who threaten suicide never commit it. In fact, it has long been known that persons who commit suicide do communicate their intention in advance—often to a therapist or physician (Shneidman & Ortega, 1969). Shneidman, Farberow, and Litman (1970) emphasized the importance of recognizing and quantitatively evaluating both *perturbation* and *lethality* in assessing suicidal risk. It is important to continue this evaluation during the course of psychotherapy, and to be wary of sudden changes in either characteristic. When the topic of suicide is rendered explicit, it may well become the center of much struggle between the therapist and the client. The best rule for the therapist is simply to persevere and never to accept the client's proposition that death would be the best solution to his or her problem.

THE RIGHT TO DIE

Sooner or later the psychotherapist working with depressed clients will be challenged on his or her right to interfere with someone else's right to die. At present, this question has become quite politicized (West, 1993). Some civil libertarians contend seriously that the right to take one's own life is precious and that mental health professionals have no authority to intervene. Needless to say, depressed clients will sometimes present the same argument. The mental health professions are not of one mind on this matter.

It is especially important to distinguish the theoretical exercise of the right to die from the clinical understanding of how powerful the desire to live really is in people if they are mentally well. If someone truly wants to die, it is not that hard to kill oneself; every year many people jump off buildings, fatally shoot themselves, or overdose on sedatives. Modern suicide prevention enterprises try to hinder such acts — and many can be prevented.

Suicidal ideation may be a symptom of a psychiatric illness or of the depression that can accompany severe physical illness, disability, bereavement, or even giving birth to a child. It may not be a positive desire to die, but rather a desire for relief from physical or psychological suffering — an escape from mental pain or what Shneidman (1993) called "psychache." If communicated, it may be a "cry for help" or reassurance. Therefore, when a patient asks his or her doctor or therapist for assistance in dying, it may well be a disguised plea for help and should be viewed as a chance to intervene. Such a patient may well change his or her mind and decide to live if provided with firm, but compassionate, intervention, which may of course include medication as well as other methods. In my experience, almost without exception, patients whom I have prevented from committing suicide have thanked me for it afterward. This holds true not only for those suffering from primary depressive disorders, but also for patients with chronic physical illnesses, such as malignancy, severe cardiac or pulmonary disease, and acquired immuno-deficiency syndrome (AIDS).

With regard to terminally ill patients, special attention should be paid to their physical and psychological comfort. It is certainly possible to keep almost anyone free of severe pain with modern treatment methods. In fact, many patients who refuse life-sustaining treatment do so not because they seek relief from intolerable pain and suffering, but because they see no other way to end their total dependence on others. Today, most Americans die in hospitals or nursing homes, where they are surrounded by assorted monitors, respirators, strange gadgets, and unfamiliar people. Rarely does the patient have any choice about the institutional environment. An alternative to hospitals and nursing homes is hospice care, which has emerged out of an awareness that the needs of the dying often are not adequately met by most modern medical institutions. Hospice care in the United States has yet to find its proper place or to be widely accepted as an essential facet of the health care delivery system. When it is, requests for assisted suicides by terminal patients will decline. In the meantime, more doctors and therapists should learn how to help people live with dignity and serenity right up to the final moments preceding death.

PSYCHOTHERAPY FOR BEREAVEMENT, MOURNING, AND GRIEF

It would be a mistake to exclude painful depressive reactions to life's real losses from a discussion of therapeutic approaches to depression. Every symptom of depressive illness, from the mildest to the most severe, can be manifested in certain cases of bereavement. Several studies (Helsing & Szklo, 1981; Parkes, 1970; Rahe, 1972) have revealed the profound psychophysiologic impact of grief. Illness, accident, suicide, or death due to any cause are far more likely to occur during the year following bereavement than would be expected in a less stressful year in the life of that person at that age. Abrupt loss, especially by violence, is particularly traumatic for the survivors. Other real losses in specific life situations may precipitate acute depression nearly indistinguishable from the grief of bereavement. The loss of a highly valued position, one's business, or one's money can lead to a suicidal grief reaction. The therapeutic approach in such cases is not dissimilar from that for treatment of depressive reactions in bereaved adults.

Psychotherapy for grief reactions, although usually brief, is not always as limited as one might expect. Many of these depressions last a full year, or even longer. Treatment should be based on the principles described previously but with certain special considerations and areas of emphasis. Some of these are listed below.

Acceptance of mourning:

It is important for the therapist to give the client permission to continue grieving and to help him or her accept grief as a natural reaction. Yet, the fact that such a reaction is natural, and thus has its own natural course, does not obviate the desirability of or need for professional help. (The analogy of childbearing — another natural, but painful, process that requires medical attention — may be helpful in explaining this to the client who berates himself or herself for needing help.) Suffering can be modified, the course abbreviated, complications prevented, and the aftermath made healthier. Reassurance that mourning is natural should include reassurance that, in time, the worst of the suffering will pass.

Acceptance of the Cessation of Mourning:

A counterpart to the therapist giving permission to grieve is giving permission to improve, with reassurance that recovery does not signify lack of a true sense of loss or of a genuine devotion to the lost person. Feeling well again does not betray the memory of the departed.

Other Aspects of the Psychotherapy for Grief Reactions:

As in the case of other depressive illnesses, psychotherapists may have a grieving client referred to them only after he or she has first been managed by other helpers. Sometimes, the therapist finds that various medications have been prescribed to sedate the newly bereaved. One of the most useful strategies in such cases is to consult the well-meaning prescribing physician so that the psychotropic medications can be discontinued. This way, the client's current drug-free state of mind can be evaluated. I have often seen apparent grief reactions improve rapidly with the discontinuation of chemicals such as benzodiazepines, which themselves have a depressing effect.

The real work of psychotherapy in grief reactions must explore and analyze in considerable detail the relationship of the bereaved to the lost person and how that relationship fits in with the rest of his or her life. For example, the living often feel a sense of guilt toward the dead. This seems to stem in part from the sense of relief at finding oneself still alive, regardless of how the loved one died. Also, the termination of an expensive, inconvenient, and painful illness may provide relief for the watchers as well as for the dying person. Gentle, nonjudgmental guidance by the therapist into these areas of feeling, together with the therapist's acceptance and even a statement that such conflicting emotions are to be expected, frequently suffices to provide some relief. However, it will often prove necessary to cover these areas repeatedly.

DEPRESSION AND AGGRESSION

It has long been accepted as a general rule that many depressed clients suffer from hostility that they have somehow turned against the self instead of directing it against the appropriate object. Indeed, revenge is a motive for some suicides, although probably no more so than hopelessness, desire for escape, or desire for reunion with a departed loved one. Karl Menninger (1978) once noted that every suicide is half a murder, meaning that persons filled with rage may turn it against themselves. In fact, many acts of violent aggression are acts of despair (Lion, 1972). A study by West (1965) revealed that in Great Britain, over a period of 20 years, approximately one third of all murderers ended up killing themselves. In Denmark, the figure was 40%.

In 1975 in Los Angeles, 10%–20% of persons who called the Suicide Prevention Center were seeking help for impulses to commit murder, not suicide (Litman, personal communication, 1975). Many others were not sure whether they wanted to kill themselves, others, or both. The implications here for the psychotherapy for depression are considerable. Therapists are well-advised to include work on both passivity and aggressiveness in their transactions with depressed clients; however, they should avoid the basic assumption that it is necessarily beneficial to encourage clients to express hostility other than that which comes naturally as integration proceeds.

TERMINATION OF THERAPY

The integrative psychotherapy for depression should not be indefinite, much less interminable. Like the interpersonal psychotherapy of Klerman and co-workers (1984), it is generally focused and time limited. However, the therapist-client relationship is bound to be a powerful therapeutic influence, regardless of the treatment method, and this relationship must be wisely employed according to each client's individual needs. It will often prove advisable to discontinue psychotherapy gradually rather than abruptly, using the client's own perception of his or her need for contact as a guide. Sometimes, formal termination of treatment is best postponed indefinitely, with the client given to understand that the therapist can be called at any time in case of need. Such calls, even once a year, may serve a very useful purpose in helping the formerly depressed client remain well.

REFERENCES

Helsing, K. J., & Szklo, M. (1981). Mortality after bereavement. *Epidemiological Review, 114*, 41.

Klerman, G. L., Weissman, M. W., Rounsaville, B. J., & Chevron, E. S. (1984). *Interpersonal psychotherapy of depression.* New York: Basic Books.

Lion, J. R. (1972). The role of depression in the treatment of aggressive personality disorders. *American Journal of Psychiatry, 129,* 347–349.

Menninger, K. A. (1978). *Man against himself.* New York: Harcourt Brace.

Parkes, C. M. (1970). The first year of bereavement: A long study of the reaction of London widows to the death of their husbands. *Psychiatry, 33,* 444–467.

Rahe, R. H. (1972). Subjects' recent life changes and their near-future illness reports. *Annals of Clinical Research, 4,* 250–265.

Robinson, L. A., Berman, J. S., & Neimeyer, R. A. (1990). Psychotherapy for the treatment of depression: A comprehensive review of controlled outcome research. *Psychological Bulletin, 108,* 30–49.

Shneidman, E. S. (1993). Suicide as psychache. *Journal of Nervous and Mental Disorders, 181,* 147–149.

Shneidman, E. S., Farberow, N., & Litman, R. (1970). *The psychology of suicide.* New York: Science House.

Shneidman, E. S., & Ortega, M. J. (Eds). (1969). *Aspects of depression.* Boston: Little, Brown & Co.

Sotsky, S. M., et al. (1991). Patient predictors of response to psychotherapy and pharmacotherapy: Findings in the NIMH Treatment of Depression Collaborative Research Program. *American Journal of Psychiatry, 148,* 997–1008.

Starvynski, A., & Greenberg, D. (1992). The psychological management of depression. *Acta Psychiatrica Scandinavica, 85,* 407–414.

West, D. J. (1965). *Murder followed by suicide.* Cambridge, MA: Harvard University Press.

West, L. J. (1975). Integrative psychotherapy of depressive illness. In F. F. Flach & S. C. Draghi (Eds.), *The nature and treatment of depression* (pp. 161–181). New York: John Wiley & Sons.

West, L. J. (1993). Reflections on the right to die. In A. Leenaars, P. Cantor, R. Litman, & R. Maris (Eds.), *Suicidology: Essays in honor of Edwin S. Shneidman* (pp. 359–376). Northvale, NJ: Jason Aronson.

8

Cognitive Therapy for Depression

Robin B. Jarrett, PhD, and A. John Rush, MD

Dr. Jarrett is Associate Professor of Psychiatry, Department of Psychiatry at the University of Texas Southwestern Medical Center, Dallas, TX. Dr. Rush is Betty Jo Hay Professor of Psychiatry, Department of Psychiatry at the University of Texas Southwestern Medical Center, Dallas, TX.

KEY POINTS

- Cognitive therapy is an effective approach for treating a subset of nonpyschotic, unipolar depressed adult outpatients.

- Three elements have been deemed essential to the psychopathology of depression: the cognitive triad, silent assumptions, and logical errors.

- Some of the processes and techniques of cognitive therapy include: developing a rapport with the patient and establishing a "collaborative alliance"; self-monitoring by the patient; patient evaluation of the validity of cognitions; and homework tailored to address the automatic thoughts, silent assumptions, or particular symptom targets chosen by the patient and the therapist.

- Based on the literature to date, cognitive therapy has been found to be at least as effective as the standard treatment (i.e., pharmacotherapy) in reducing depressive symptoms of outpatients suffering from unipolar major depressive disorder.

- Further study on the cognitive model is necessary to determine the conditions under which cognitive therapy is maximally effective and whether such therapy reduces relapse or recurrence after the acute phase or in the continuation/maintenance phase.

INTRODUCTION

Cognitive therapy is a short-term psychosocial intervention designed both to ameliorate the symptoms of nonpsychotic, unipolar depression (i.e., it is designed for symptom reduction) and to decrease the probability that depression will recur (i.e., it is designed for prophylaxis). This chapter briefly describes the cognitive model of depression, the typical course of cognitive therapy, and the evidence for its effectiveness.

THE COGNITIVE MODEL

The premise of the cognitive model is that cognitions (images and thoughts) influence emotions and behaviors. This premise is grounded in a phenomenological approach to psychology, which assumes that behavior is influenced by the person's perception of himself or herself and of the world. According to the cognitive model, the central feature of depression is a group of distorted cognitions. Therefore, within the cognitive model, other symptoms typical of depression, such as motivational deficits, suicidal impulses, and sadness, are augmented by distorted thinking patterns.

Cognitive Therapy's Unit of Focus — Distorted Cognitions:

Rush (1983) defined cognitions as images and thoughts or "what a person thinks to himself in a situation." According to the cognitive model, cognitions are important because they are related to the feelings and behavior that occur in the situation. Beck (1963) maintained that the cognitions associated with depression are automatic, involuntary, plausible, persistent, and often contain a theme of loss. He distinguished between socially accepted or objective definitions of particular events (e.g., loss) and private meanings of events (i.e., the significance of the event to the person). Beck stressed that it is the private interpretation of events that is critical to the emotional responses that follow them. The emphasis on the private meanings of events reflects the roots of cognitive therapy in phenomenological conceptualization of psychopathology. However, it is also the disparity between private and public meanings of events that result in discrimination between "distorted" and "rational" cognitions.

In describing and theorizing about depression, Beck (1967, 1972, 1976) deemed three elements essential to the psychopathology of depression: the cognitive triad, silent assumptions, and logical errors.

Cognitive Triad:

The cognitive triad consists of the negative views that depressed persons hold about themselves, their world, and their future (Table 8.1). Generally, they assume that they, their

---

Table 8.1
EXAMPLES OF COGNITIONS FROM THE AUTOMATIC THOUGHTS QUESTIONNAIRE

I feel like I'm up against the world.
I'm no good.
Why can't I ever succeed?
No one understands me.
I've let people down.
I don't think I can go on.
I wish I were a better person.
I'm so weak.
My life's not going the way I want it to.
I'm so disappointed in myself.
Nothing feels good anymore.
I can't stand this anymore.
I can't get started.

Source: Hollon, S. D., Kendall, P. C. (1980). Cognitive self-statements in depression: Development of an automatic thoughts questionnaire. *Cognitive Therapy Research, 4,* 383-395. Reprinted with permission from Plenum Publishing Corp.

world, and their future lack some feature(s) that is a prerequisite for happiness. For example, depressed clients may view themselves as unworthy, inadequate, or incompetent. They may view their environment as continually demanding and unsupporting. They may describe the future as hopeless and predict that their deficits and current pain will continue indefinitely. These negative views account for, maintain, or contribute to other symptoms commonly found in the depressive syndrome. That is, if depressed people think that "today will be just as miserable as yesterday," they will feel and behave as if this thought were literally true or valid. For example, they may feel sad and stay in bed. These negative views are called *automatic thoughts*; they are found in the stream of consciousness of the depressed person in specific situations.

Silent Assumptions:

The second element found in the psychopathology of depression consists of silent assumptions or rules. These are inarticulated rules that influence the emotional, behavioral, and thinking patterns of the depressed client (Table 8.2). Silent assumptions are psychological constructs on which the client bases his or her emotional and behavioral responses. For example, the depressed client may believe, "If I am not loved by everyone, I'm unworthy." These stable beliefs develop from early experience and subsequently influence the client's responses to events. According to the cognitive model, these silent assumptions give rise to automatic thoughts. Silent assumptions are typically stated as "if-then" premises that can be identified by examining patterns within a group of automatic thoughts or behavioral responses.

Depressive assumptions are typically inferred by examining the situation, emotions, and themes associated with the array of negative automatic thoughts. For example, a depressed woman may report sadness when her husband does not compliment her on her appearance. She may report think-

---

Table 8.2
SAMPLE ITEMS FROM THE DYSFUNCTIONAL ATTITUDES SCALE

It is difficult to be happy unless one is good looking, intelligent, rich, and creative.

Happiness is more a matter of my attitude toward myself than the way other people feel about me.

People will probably think less of me if I make a mistake.

If I do not do well all the time, people will not respect me.

Taking even a small risk is foolish because the loss is likely to be a disaster.

It is possible to gain another person's respect without being especially talented at anything.

I cannot be happy unless most people I know admire me.

If a person asks for help, it is a sign of weakness.

---

ing, "He is not attracted to me anymore because I am ugly." She may also report feeling dysphoric when a friend talks to her for only 5 minutes in the grocery store. She may report thinking, "She would want to spend more time with me if I weren't so dull." Through repeated examples and verbal exchange, the therapist and client may infer the silent assumption, "If others don't attend to me, it's: (a) something to be disturbed about and (b) because of a deficit I have."

The cognitive model posits that these inappropriate assumptions are activated more frequently than appropriate (undistorted) assumptions when a person is depressed. It is assumed that as the depression becomes more severe, the client's thinking becomes more disparate despite logical or objective evidence to the contrary.

Logical Errors:

The third element essential to this cognitive model are the logical errors spawned by the negative automatic thoughts made by the depressed client. Logical errors are identified by examining logical relationships between a specific event and the associated negative automatic thought. Some examples of logical errors include: arbitrary inference, selective attention, overgeneralization, magnification or minimization, and personalization. Arbitrary inference occurs when the depressed client draws conclusions that are not supported by logical or environmental data. Selective attention refers to emphasizing certain details and ignoring others. Overgeneralization includes drawing conclusions about one's ability, performance, or worth based on a single incident. Magnification or minimization refers to exaggerating or diminishing, respectively, the importance of an event. Personalization involves associating events with oneself when logic or data would prohibit such associations.

The Vulnerability For and Maintenance of Depression:

According to Beck and Greenberg (1976), the existence of silent assumptions increases a client's vulnerability or predisposition to depression. These assumptions may develop through interactions with significant others. In particular, depressive assumptions are learned in the context of "an unfavorable life situation," such as the loss of a parent or chronic rejection by peers. Later in life, when the person is exposed to a situation analogous to the original unfavorable life situation, he or she employs the previously learned assumptions.

Once activated, these schemata or assumptions are applied to an ever-widening array of stimulus situations and thereby lead to more negative automatic thinking. For example, a person who is overly concerned with approval from others may view normal day-to-day transactions as if they meant he or she is not liked by anyone (e.g., the flight attendant on the airplane didn't smile. That means, "no one likes me.")

The typical emotional, motivational, behavioral, and vegetative depressive symptoms (e.g., hopelessness, apathy, agitation, and sleep disturbance (are made worse by this negative automatic thinking. As depressive symptoms worsen, the distorted thinking increases. Beck and colleagues (1979) termed the relationship between depressive symptoms and thoughts a "vicious cycle," a "circular feedback model," and the "downward spiral of depression."

THE TYPICAL COURSE OF COGNITIVE THERAPY

Establishing a Therapeutic Alliance and Rationale:

One of the first steps in cognitive therapy involves developing a rapport with the client and establishing a *collaborative alliance*. The therapist's role in this alliance is to guide the client. For example, each session begins with the therapist and client listing and prioritizing items on the "agenda" to be covered. The competent cognitive therapist not only has refined general psychotherapeutic skills (i.e., he or she is perceived as warm, genuine, empathic, and able to understand and reflect the client's thinking), but also can remain objective and logical about the automatic thoughts and emotional responses that are identified. The therapist usually phrases most comments as questions, to be answered by the client, rather than as statements. The cognitive therapist typically avoids attempting to "persuade" the client that his or her thoughts are dysfunctional. Instead, the therapist encourages the client to test the objectivity or validity of specific thoughts or ideas by examining their inherent logic and/or by seeking supportive or discomfirming data within the client's daily life. Such an alliance has been labeled *collaborative empiricism* (Beck et al., 1979).

The therapeutic alliance is of special importance when

working with depressed clients, who characteristically overpersonalize and are likely to respond negatively to neutral or even positive interpersonal interactions. When problems occur within the therapeutic context (e.g., relationship difficulties, or missed appointments), these problems are conceptualized within the cognitive model; that is, corresponding thoughts and emotions are identified and problem-solving strategies implemented. For instance, a depressed client may report missing a therapy session after thinking, "I've been depressed before and received therapy. I'm depressed again, so this won't work either." The therapist can consider the report of these thoughts as an opportunity to review the (a) similarities and dissimilarities of past and current therapies, (b) evidence supporting or refuting the notion that cognitive therapy will not work, (c) advantages and disadvantages of cognitive therapy to date, and (d) changes that may need to be made in the therapy.

To foster a collaborative alliance, much time is devoted to providing a rationale for treatment. The verbal rationale may be supplemented by asking the client to read Beck and Greenberg's *Coping With Depression* (1976). This pamphlet aids in "socializing" the client to cognitive therapy by (a) describing many of the depressive symptoms from which the client may suffer, (b) illustrating dysfunctional thinking, (c) focusing on the relationship between dysfunctional thinking and depression, and (d) encouraging the client that his or her problems can be alleviated by learning to recognize negative thoughts, testing the validity of the thoughts, and problem solving.

PROCESSES AND TECHNIQUES OF COGNITIVE THERAPY

Self-Monitoring:

Self-monitoring is used to aid clients in identifying thoughts that accompany uncomfortable emotions and difficult situations. Through completion of the Daily Record of Dysfunctional Thoughts (Table 8.3) and dialogue, the client begins to distinguish and to note the relationship between thoughts, events, emotions, and other behaviors. For example, a client

---

Table 8.3
DAILY RECORD OF DYSFUNCTIONAL THOUGHTS

Situation
Describe:
1. Actual event leading up to unpleasant emotion, or
2. Stream of thoughts, daydream, or recollection, leading to unpleasant emotion.

Emotion(s)
1. Specify sad/anxious/angry, etc.
2. Rate degree of emotion, 1–100.

Automatic Thought(s)
1. Write automatic thought(s) that preceded emotion(s).
2. Rate belief in automatic thought(s), 0%–100%.

Rational Response
1. Write rational response to automatic thought(s).
2. Rate belief in rational response, 0%–100%.

Outcome
1. Rerate belief in automatic thought(s), 0%–100%.
2. Specify and rate subsequent emotions, 0%–100%.

Explanation
When you experience an unpleasant emotion, note the situation that seemed to stimulate the emotion. (If the emotion occurred while you were thinking, daydreaming, etc., please note this.) Then note the automatic thought associated with the emotion. Record the degree to which you believe this thought: 0%=not at all; 100%=completely. In rating degree of emotion: 1=trace; 100=the most intense possible.

Source: Beck, A. T., et al. (1979). *Cognitive therapy of depression.* New York: Guilford Press. Reprinted with permission from Guilford Press.

may note that he or she feels sad (i.e., the emotion) when a co-worker does not say, "Good morning" (i.e., the situation), and he or she thinks, "Nobody likes me here enough to say hello" (i.e., the automatic thought). After noticing the covariation between this situation, emotion, and thought, it is understandable that the client avoids the office coffee break; that is, he or she assumes nobody likes him or her.

After clients have learned self-monitoring, they are taught to identify themes, ideas that recur across situations, by reviewing past records and sessions (e.g., fearing rejection, seeking approval). By identifying and discussing these pervasive themes, clients and therapists infer the clients' general rules or silent assumptions.

Table 8.4
BEHAVIORAL TECHNIQUES

Activity Scheduling

Mastery and Pleasure Ratings

Graded Task Assignment

Cognitive Rehearsal

Assertive Training/Role Playing

Mood Graph

Source: Rush, A. J. (1983). Cognitive therapy of depression: Rationale, techniques, and efficacy. *Psychiatric Clinics of North America, 6,* 105-127. Reprinted with permission from W. B. Saunders Company.

Evaluating the Validity of Cognitions:

Subsequently, clients learn to determine the extent to which their cognitions (i.e., automatic thoughts and silent assumptions) correspond to an objective appraisal of their situation. When the thoughts or assumptions do not match the "evidence," clients are taught to revise these cognitions with more accurate ones and to carry out responses that are consistent with this modified view.

The general process of evaluating the validity of automatic thoughts or silent assumptions is accomplished through a variety of techniques (Tables 8.4 and 8.5). When evaluating the validity of cognitions, the first basic goal is to teach clients to recognize that thoughts and beliefs are inferences about the world rather than facts. When clients can conceptualize thoughts as assumptions or hypotheses rather than as facts, they can develop some "distance" from the emotions accompanying the thoughts. Hence, clients learn to scrutinize their thoughts by asking questions such as: What part of my situation is a fact and what part is my belief? What evidence is there to support or to refute my thoughts? What are some alternative explanations for my thoughts? How would a nondepressed person view my situation? Even if my thoughts match the facts, is it truly as bad as it seems? Through this type of questioning, clients learn to recognize and to correct logical errors.

Table 8.5
COGNITIVE TECHNIQUES

Recording Automatic Thoughts (Cognitions)

Reattribution Techniques

Responding to Negative Cognitions

Counting Automatic Thoughts

Identifying Assumptions

Modifying Shoulds

Pro-Con Refutation of Assumptions

Homework to Test Old Assumptions

Homework to Test New Assumptions

Source: Rush, A. J. (1983). Cognitive therapy of depression. Rationale, techniques, and efficacy. *Psychiatric Clinics of North America, 6,* 105-127. Reprinted with permission from W. B. Saunders Company.

In addition to learning to evaluate their thoughts logically, clients learn to view these thoughts as hypotheses that can be tested. They learn to (a) state their cognitions in a testable form (i.e., make a prediction); (b) arrange and implement a test of the prediction; (c) record the results; (d) compare the results with the prediction; and (e) query whether additional experiments are necessary to test the validity of the thought. For example, a depressed lawyer reported, "I'm so disorganized and distracted, I'll never complete my work." Such a prediction is especially suited to a common technique used in cognitive therapy called graded task assignment. Through graded task assignment, the client was taught to operationalize work (e.g., a legal report) and to break it down into small, specific, realistic tasks to be completed over time. Within the experiment, the lawyer predicted she could not even complete the first step of gathering the related legal books and moving all other distracting materials from the desk. The therapist identified the thoughts that might interfere with the task (e.g., "I'm too incompetent to complete the first step"), and emphasized partial successes. Each component of completing the legal report was specified, and accomplishing the tasks was viewed as an experiment. Throughout the experiment, the client recorded her progress and compared these results with her initial prediction. At the end of the experiment, the client concluded that she was, in fact, able to make some progress on her legal report and had made overly pessimistic predictions that interfered with her working effectively.

Homework:

One of the most important aspects of cognitive therapy is the "homework" assignment that is completed outside of the therapeutic session. Homework is tailored to address the automatic thoughts, silent assumptions, or particular symptom targets chosen by both the client and the therapist. Each session includes a review of the homework. Noncompliance, and any other difficult behavior affecting homework assignments, is dealt with using a cognitive model, inquiring, for example, as to what thoughts and emotions occurred to the client when he or she had difficulty beginning the homework. For an illustration of a homework assignment, refer to Table 8.3.

Frequency, Length, and Modality of Treatment:

To date, few studies are designed to determine what, if any, relationship exists between the frequency or length of treatment and response to cognitive therapy. One preliminary report suggested that moderately to severely depressed clients evidence fewer dropouts and greater reduction in symptoms when treated twice a week than when treated once a week (Beck et al., 1979). In research protocols, cognitive therapy typically takes place twice a week for 10 to 16 weeks, for a total of 20 sessions. Experienced cognitive therapists recommend that the frequency of the sessions be determined by the severity of the depression; as severity increases, frequency increases.

No published controlled studies to date have examined the effect of maintenance or "booster" sessions on the therapeutic response of clients who have been diagnosed with recurrent depression. In practice, it is common for clients to participate in booster sessions (once or twice a month) for 6–12 months after routine cognitive therapy.

The typical modality in which cognitive therapy occurs is individual sessions. Rush and Watkins (1981) compared cognitive therapy administered to an individual with a group setting and found an advantage for the individual modality. Clinical experience suggests that cognitive therapy can also be used with couples (Rush, Shaw, & Khatami, 1980).

THE EFFECTIVENESS OF COGNITIVE THERAPY

There is ample evidence that the acute phase of cognitive

therapy reduces depressive symptoms. Jarrett and Maguire (1991) and Jarrett and Down (in press) reviewed and abstracted the literature from 1967 to 1990. Other reviews of the literature include Jarrett and Rush (1986, 1994), Dobson (1989), Shaw (1989), and Wilson (1989). In general, the results can be summarized by concluding that cognitive therapy, whether used alone or in combination with antidepressant medication, reduces depressive symptoms during the acute phase. When researchers compared cognitive therapy with behavior therapy (Gallagher & Thompson, 1982; Thompson, Gallagher, & Breckenridge, 1987) or interpersonal psychotherapy (Elkin et al., 1989), they generally found no statistically significant differences; these short-term psychotherapies all reduce depressive symptoms. Similarly, when researchers (Blackburn et al., 1981; Elkin et al., 1989; Murphy et al., 1984) compared cognitive therapy used alone with pharmacotherapy used alone, they did not find any significant differences in reducing depressive symptoms. However, Rush and colleagues (1977) and Blackburn and co-workers (1981), when confining their results to referrals from the general practice clinic, reported that cognitive therapy alone reduced depressive symptoms more than pharmacotherapy alone.

The combination of cognitive therapy with pharmacotherapy typically does not reduce depressive symptoms more than cognitive therapy used alone (Beck et al., 1985; Blackburn et al., 1981 [general practice participants only]; Covi & Lipman, 1987; Murphy et al., 1984; Rush & Watkins, 1981). One exception to these data is the finding by Blackburn and co-workers (1981) where the combination of cognitive therapy plus pharmacotherapy reduced depressive symptoms more than cognitive therapy used alone in treating psychiatric clinic outpatients. In summary, based on the literature to date, cognitive therapy has been found to be at least as effective as the standard treatment (i.e., pharmacotherapy) in reducing depressive symptoms of outpatients suffering from unipolar major depressive disorder.

Conclusions regarding the prophylactic value of cognitive

therapy in reducing depressive relapse/recurrences are premature. In general, the research can be summarized by stating that the relapse/recurrence rate 1 year after completing the acute phase of cognitive therapy has ranged from 0% (Simons, Murphy, Levine, & Wetzel, 1986) to 50% (Kovacs, Rush, Beck & Hollon, 1981). Methodological problems complicate this literature because the studies were designed to investigate the effectiveness of the acute phase of cognitive therapy rather than the prophylactic effect of cognitive therapy. Promising results have been obtained by Blackburn, Eunson, and Bishop (1986), who suggested the cumulative probability of recurrence was 23%. However, more research is certainly needed in this area.

Predicting Response to Cognitive Therapy:

At present, no definitive predictors of response to cognitive therapy exist. To date, the literature on indications for cognitive therapy should be viewed as hypotheses needing further testing rather than as conclusions ready to guide clinical practice. However, several clinically interesting findings are worthy of further study. For example, pretreatment symptom severity appears to be an important indication for cognitive therapy. Clients with fewer symptoms may show a better response (Beckham, 1989; Elkin et al., 1989; Neimeyer & Weiss, 1990; Simons et al., 1985). It is noteworthy that although clinicians frequently select treatment modalities based on the extent to which depressed clients have endogenous or nonendogenous symptom profiles, little research has been conducted suggesting that clients with a nonendogenous or endogenous symptom profile respond better or worse to cognitive therapy (Blackburn et al., 1981; Kovacs et al., 1981). The presence of a personality disorder (Thompson, Gallagher, & Czirr, 1988) or marital discord (Jacobson, Holtzworth-Munroe, & Schmaling, 1989) appears to complicate the response to cognitive therapy when delivered in its typical format.

Finally, Beck and colleagues (1979) stated that clients with hallucinations, delusions, organic brain syndrome, borderline personality disorder, and schizoaffective disorders may respond poorly when cognitive therapy is conducted in its typical time-limited format. Failure in treating depression with cognitive therapy has been the subject of review by Rush and Shaw (1983). New directions for research on cognitive therapy include adapting cognitive therapy to treat outpatients with recurrent major depression (Jarrett, 1992), depressed children and adolescents (Wilkes & Rush, 1988), depressed inpatients (Thase & Wright, 1991), and pharmacologically stabilized clients with bipolar depression.

CONCLUSION

Cognitive therapy is an effective approach for treating a subset of nonpsychotic, unipolar depressed adult outpatients. To date, the literature suggests that cognitive therapy reduces depressive symptoms in this subgroup. Whether cognitive therapy reduces relapse or recurrence after the acute phase or in the continuation/maintenance phase remains a subject requiring further study. Theoretically, it is unclear through what mechanisms cognitive therapy produces its effects and to what extent the cognitive model accurately describes the development and maintenance of depression. Practical issues involving the conditions under which cognitive therapy is maximally effective are yet to be resolved. These questions include when to combine cognitive therapy with antidepressant pharmacotherapy, what are the most effective and efficient modalities for delivering cognitive therapy, and which clients are most likely to respond to this treatment.

REFERENCES

Beck, A. T. (1963). Thinking and depression: Idiosyncratic content and cognitive distortion. *Archives of General Psychiatry, 9*, 324–333.

Beck, A. T. (1967). *Depression: Clinical, experimental, and theoretical aspects.* New York: Harper & Row.

Beck, A. T. (1972). *Depression: Causes and treatment.* Philadelphia: University of Pennsylvania Press.

Beck, A. T. (1976). *Cognitive therapy and the emotional disorders.* New York: International Universities Press.

Beck, A. T., et al. (1979). *Cognitive therapy of depression.* New York: Guilford Press.

Beck, A. T., et al. (1985). Treatment of depression with cognitive therapy and amitriptyline. *Archives of General Psychiatry, 42*, 142–145.

Beck, A. T., & Greenberg, R. (1976). *Coping with depression.* Philadelphia: Center for Cognitive Therapy.

Beckham, E. E. (1989). Improvement after evaluation in psychotherapy of depression: Evidence of a placebo effect? *Journal of Clinical Psychology, 45*, 945–950.

Blackburn, I. M., et al. (1981). The efficacy of cognitive therapy in depression: A treatment trial using cognitive therapy and pharmacotherapy, each alone and in combination. *British Journal of Psychiatry, 139*, 181–189.

Blackburn, I. M., Eunson, K. M., & Bishop, S. (1986). A two-year naturalistic follow-up of depressed patients treated with cognitive therapy, pharmacotherapy, and a combination of both. *Journal of Affective Disorders, 10*, 67–75.

Covi, L., & Lipman, R. S. (1987). Cognitive behavioral group psychotherapy combined with imipramine in major depression. *Psychopharmacology Bulletin, 23*, 173–176.

Dobson, K. S. (1989). A meta-analysis of the efficacy of cognitive therapy for depression. *Journal of Consulting and Clinical Psychology, 57,* 414–419.

Elkin, I., et al. (1989). National Institute of Mental Health Treatment of Depression Collaborative Research Program. General effectiveness of treatments. *Archives of General Psychiatry, 46,* 971–982.

Gallagher, D.E., & Thompson, L. W. (1982). Treatment of major depressive disorder in older adult outpatients with brief psychotherapies. *Psychotherapy: Theory, Research, and Practice, 19,* 482–489.

Jacobson, N. S., Holtzworth-Munroe, A., & Schmaling, K. B. (1989). Marital therapy and spouse involvement in the treatment of depression, agoraphobia, and alcoholism. *Journal of Consulting and Clinical Psychology, 57,* 5–10.

Jarrett, R. B. (1992). *Cognitive therapy for recurrent unipolar major depressive disorder: The continuation/maintenance phase.* Unpublished manuscript.

Jarrett, R. B., & Down, M. (in press). Psychotherapy for adults with major depressive disorder. In *Clinical practice guideline no. 5: Detection, diagnosis, and treatment of depression* (chap. 10). Agency for Health Care Policy and Research. Rockville, MD: National Technical Information Service.

Jarrett, R. B., & Maguire, M. A. (1991). *Short-term psychotherapy for depression.* Unpublished manuscipt. Technical review commissioned by the Agency for Health Care Policy and Research Depression Guideline Panel.

Jarrett, R. B., & Rush, A. J. (1986). Psychotherapeutic approaches for depression. In J. O. Cavenar (Ed.), *Psychiatry* (pp. 1–35). Philadelphia: J. B. Lippincott.

Jarret, R. B., & Rush, A. J. (1994). Short-term psychotherapy of depression disorders: Current status and future directions. *Psychiatry, 57,* 115–132.

Kovacs, M., Rush, A. J., Beck, A. T., & Hollon, S. D. (1981). Depressed outpatients treated with cognitive therapy or pharmacotherapy: A one-year follow-up. *Archives of General Psychiatry, 38,* 33–41.

Murphy, G. E., et al. (1984). Cognitive therapy and pharmacotherapy: Singly and together in the treatment of depression. *Archives of General Psychiatry, 41*, 33–41.

Neimeyer, R. A., & Weiss, M. E. (1990). Cognitive and symptomatic predictors of outcome of group therapies for depression. *Journal of Cognitive Psychotherapy: An International Quarterly, 4*, 23–32.

Rush, A. J. (1983). Cognitive therapy of depression: Rationale, techniques, and efficacy. *Psychiatric Clinics of North America, 6*, 105–127.

Rush, A. J., et al. (1977). Comparative efficacy of cognitive therapy and pharmacotherapy in the treatment of depressed outpatients. *Cognitive Therapy Research, 1*, 17–37.

Rush, A. J., & Shaw, B. F. (1983). Failures in treating depression by cognitive behavior therapy. In E. B. Foa, & P. M. G. Emmelkamp (Eds.), *Failures in behavior therapy* (pp. 213–224). New York: John Wiley & Sons.

Rush, A. J., Shaw, B. F., & Khatami, M. (1980). Cognitive therapy of depression: Utilizing the couples system. *Cognitive Therapy Research, 4*, 103–113.

Rush, A. J., & Watkins, J. T. (1981). Group versus individual cognitive therapy: A pilot study. *Cognitive Therapy Research, 5*, 95–103.

Shaw, B. F. (1989). Cognitive-behavior therapies for major depression: Current status with an emphasis on prophylaxis. *Psychiatric Journal of the University of Ottawa, 14*, 403–408.

Simons, A. D., et al. (1985). Predicting response to cognitive therapy of depression: The role of learned resourcefulness. *Cognitive Therapy Research, 9*, 79–89.

Simons, A. D., Murphy, G. E., Levine J. L., & Wetzel, R. D. (1986). Cognitive therapy and pharmacotherapy for depression. *Archives of General Psychiatry, 43*, 43–48.

Thase, M. E., & Wright, J. H. (1991). Cognitive-behavior therapy manual for depressed inpatients: A treatment protocol outline. *Behavior Therapy, 22*, 579–595.

Thompson, L. W., Gallagher, D., & Breckenridge, J. S. (1987). Comparative effectiveness of psychotherapies for depressed elders. *Journal of Consulting and Clinical Psychology, 55,* 385–390.

Thompson, L. W., Gallagher, D., & Czirr, R. (1988). Personality disorder and outcome in the treatment of late-life depression. *Journal of Geriatric Psychiatry, 21,* 133–146.

Wilkes, T. C. R., & Rush, A. J. (1988). Adaptations of cognitive therapy for depressed adolescents. *Journal of the Academy of Child and Adolescent Psychiatry, 27,* 381–386.

Wilson, P. H. (1989). Cognitive therapy for depression: Empirical findings and methodological issues in the evaluation of outcome. *Behavior Change, 6,* 85–95.

FOR FURTHER READING

Beck, A. T., & Freeman, A. (1990). *Cognitive therapy of personality disorders.* New York: Guilford Press.

Safran, J. D., & Segal, Z. V. (1990). *Interpersonal process in cognitive therapy.* New York: Basic Books.

Schyler, D. (1990). *A practical guide to cognitive therapy.* New York: Norton.

9

Behavioral Counseling for Older Adults with Depression

Duane A. Lundervold, RhD

Dr. Lundervold is a family therapist at Boone County Youth and Family Counseling, Boone County Hospital, Boone, IA.

KEY POINTS

- Older adults (i.e., adults older than 55 years of age) report as many depressive symptoms as younger adults; however, they are less likely to be diagnosed with major depressive disorder.

- Prevalence estimates of depression are presented for older adults in three settings: community dwellings, nursing homes, and hospitals.

- Late-life depression is a function of interacting bioenvironmental variables.

- Diagnosing geriatric depression requires a multidimensional approach that includes medical and cognitive evaluation, symptomatic psychiatric assessment, and behavioral analysis.

- The first functional analysis of depression, that of B. F. Skinner, has been central to all subsequent behavioral theories of depression.

- In the behavioral approach to depression, depression and reinforcement are related phenomena. *Depression* is defined as a response class of an array of behaviors that vary; *reinforcement* is defined as positive social and physical environment interactions.

- Several studies of individual and group behavioral counseling are reviewed. The results of this research validates the efficacy of behavioral counseling in older adults with major depressive disorder.

INTRODUCTION

Mental health disorders—especially depression—in older adults represent a growing concern (Aldwin, Spiro, Levenson, & Brosse, 1989; Cohen & Eisdorfer, 1988; Newman, 1989). Until recently, many mental health professionals believed that older adults would not benefit from mental health counseling. Fortunately, evidence from large-scale clinical trials suggests that the benefits of counseling older adults with depression are equal to those of younger cohorts (Gallagher-Thompson, Hanley-Peterson, & Thompson, 1990).

This chapter provides a summary of current research on behavioral counseling for older adults with depression. For the purposes of this chapter, "behavioral" is defined functionally. In doing so, controlled single-case or group-design research using self-described behavioral or cognitive-behavioral interventions for older adults with depression is included. The review focuses on the prevalence of major depressive disorder in older adults; evaluation, diagnosis, and behavioral assessment of depressed behavior; a brief description of behavioral theory regarding depressed behavior; and individual and group behavioral counseling interventions.

PREVALENCE OF GERIATRIC DEPRESSION

Older adults (those older than 55 years of age) report as many depressive symptoms as younger adults but are less likely to receive a diagnosis of major depressive disorder (Blazer & Williams, 1980). There are several possible reasons for this outcome. First, older adults may be more likely to experience mild forms of depression as opposed to severe forms. Second, the higher rate of physical illness in older adults may distort the frequency of reporting and detecting depressed behavior. Finally, some investigators suggest that current diagnostic criteria may not be "age fair," thereby resulting in an underdiagnosis of major depression in older adults (Blazer, Hughes, & George, 1987). Prevalence estimates of depression are available for older adults in three settings: community dwellings, nursing homes, and hospitals.

Community Dwellings:

Most cases of depression in older adults can be described as relapses (Weissmann & Myers, 1979). "Reported" prevalence estimates vary with the methods by which depression is defined and measured. This evidence not withstanding, depression remains one of the most prevalent behavioral disorders among older adults, occurring for the first time in 10%–20% of the population older than age 60 (Ruegg, Zisook, & Neal, 1988). The prevalence of major depression in community-dwelling older adults is 2%–4%, whereas less severe forms of dysphoria range from 5%–44% (Blazer & Williams, 1980). However, these data may underestimate the prevalence of major depressive disorders due to a failure to consider comorbid disorders. For example, recent evidence suggests that major depression and Alzheimer's disease coexist in a significant number of older adults (Blazer & Williams, 1980).

Caregivers of family members with a dementing illness appear to be at greatest risk of developing a major depressive disorder. Current evidence suggests that approximately 50% of caregivers experience major depressive disorder during the caregiving process (Teri & Wagner, 1992). There is some question as to the reliability of these data, due to the sampling procedures used (i.e., nonpopulation-based studies); nonetheless, a large proportion of caregivers develop major depressive disorder (Schulz, Visintainer, & Williamson, 1990).

Nursing Homes:

Only recently have systematic attempts been made to estimate the prevalence of behavioral disorders in nursing home residents. Recent evidence suggests that approximately 10%–14% of nursing home residents meet the *Diagnostic and Statistical Manual of Mental Disorders* (DSM-IV) criteria for major depression (American Psychiatric Association, 1994; Parmalee,

Katz, & Lawton, 1992; Rovner et al., 1990). The occurrence of comorbid depression and dementia results in another 3% of nursing home residents being diagnosed. The incidence of an episode of major depression in nursing home residents is reported to be 7.6% per year (Parmalee et al., 1992). When considering an increase in severity from minor depression (i.e., symptoms of dysphoria) to major depression, the incidence is 16.2% per year (Parmalee et al., 1992).

Hospitals:

Older adults are more likely to experience physical health problems than their younger counterparts. Of all the people older than 65 years of age, it is estimated that 85% report at least one chronic illness (Hendricks & Hendricks, 1977). Less than 20% of those who reach the seventh decade of life are free of disease (Jarvik & Perl, 1981). Underdiagnosis of depression in medically ill older adults is a frequent occurrence (Koenig, Meador, Cohen, & Blazer, 1988a). Recent studies suggest that major depressive disorder and physical illness coexist in approximately 14% of older adults (Incalzi et al., 1991; Koenig, Meador, Cohen, & Blazer, 1988b).

BIOENVIRONMENTAL ETIOLOGY

Late-life depression is a function of interacting bioenvironmental variables (Goldfried & Sprafkin, 1976; Lewin & Lundervold, 1990). In such a model, both organismic (biologic) and environmental (social and physical) factors are considered as etiologic agents that affect behavior. External factors related to the onset of depression are conceptually defined as "loss" and are related to diminished functional capacity and loss of loved objects and activities. Decreased physical functioning may make a person vulnerable to depression by way of diminished access to social reinforcers and the meaning attributed to illness/disability. Figure 9.1 presents a conceptual model of these interacting influences.

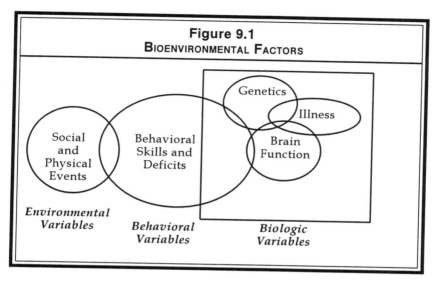

Figure 9.1
BIOENVIRONMENTAL FACTORS

Environmental events may contribute to depressed behavior as well. For example, in high-crime neighborhoods, the social environment may result in increased social isolation and decreased opportunity to engage in pleasant events. The physical structure of the environment may handicap older adults in the case of limited or inaccessible public transportation or city streets that are too wide for them to cross safely. As a result, access to social reinforcers is lost—perhaps through the death of family members and friends. Acute and chronic environmental and physiologic stressors combined with preexisting behavioral deficits to cope with such events set the stage for depressed behavior. Increased vulnerability due to biologic predisposition and behavioral deficits lower a person's threshold for coping with bioenvironmental perturbations.

DIAGNOSIS OF GERIATRIC DEPRESSION

Diagnosis of geriatric depression requires a multidimensional approach that includes medical and cognitive evaluation, symptomatic psychiatric assessment, and behavioral analysis. The complexity of geriatric depression and clinical research and practice suggest that such an approach is valuable.

Medical and Cognitive Evaluation:

Medical evaluation of physical disorders that mimic depression in older adults is critical. Prior to the initiation of counseling, the counselor should request permission to review and discuss the client's medical record with his or her physician or suggest the client undergo a physical examination to rule out biologic causes. It must also be ascertained whether other medically related factors, such as polypharmacy (the use of multiple medications), are contributing to reports of depression. Tables 9.1 and 9.2 provide examples of medications and physical illnesses that can mimic depression. With careful evaluation and medical treatment, depression caused by physical illness or iatrogenic causes can be alleviated.

Table 9.1
MEDICATIONS THAT CAN MIMIC DEPRESSION

Antihypertensives	Analgesics	Cardiovascular Agents	Antipsychotics	Sedatives/Hypnotics
Reserpine (Diupres)	Morphine	Digitalis	Chlorpromazine (Thorazine)	Barbiturates
Methyldopa (Aldomet)	Codeine	Diuretics	Haloperidol (Haldol)	Benzodiazepines
Propranolol (Inderal)	Meperidine (Demerol)	Lidocaine (Xylocaine)	Thiothixene (Navane)	Meprobamate (Miltown)
Clonidine (Catapres)	Pentazocine (Talwin)			Chloral hydrate
Hydralazine (Apresazide)	Propoxyphene (Darvon)			Flurazepam (Dalmane)

Several important reasons are evident for assessing cognitive impairment as part of a medical evaluation or separately in the context of the assessment conducted by a mental health or rehabilitation counselor. First, cognitive assessment may reveal a previously undetected cognitive impairment that may be medically treatable. Second, cognitive impairment, such as memory loss due to dementia, is an age-associated disorder and may be linked with depression. Persons with dementia and depression may also benefit from behavioral interventions for depression (Bourgeois, 1990; Teri & Uomoto, 1991). Finally, a direct relationship between an older adult's report of memory problems and cognitive impairment does not exist (Zarit, 1980). It becomes necessary to evaluate such reports more closely to determine the variables that control the reporting of such problems. Older adults who are depressed may

Table 9.2
PHYSICAL ILLNESSES THAT CAN MIMIC DEPRESSION

Neurologic	*Endocrinologic*	*Cardiovascular*	*Infections*	*Metabolic*
Parkinson's disease	Hypo-/hyper-thyroidism	Emphysema	Encephalitis	Dehydration
Brain tumor	Addison's disease	Cardiac insufficiency	Urinary tract infection	Uremia
				Hypoxia
Intercranial aneurysm	Cushing's disease	Anoxia	Meningitis	
Closed-head injury	Hyperparathyroidism	Chronic obstructive pulmonary disease	Bacterial infection	
Stroke				
Transient ischemic attacks	Diabetes mellitus			
Dementia (all types)				

also report having problems with recall and concentration. In such cases, objective memory assessment will reveal no memory deficit *per se*; rather, a slowness to respond and an attempt to avoid the task are observed. For older adults who report memory problems, treatment of depression may result in improved memory (LaRue, D'Elia, Clark, Spar, & Jarvik, 1986).

One of the more popular instruments for screening cognitive impairment is the Mini-Mental State Examination developed by Folstein and colleagues (Folstein, Folstein, & McHugh, 1975). This instrument consists of 30 questions with cutoff scores for mild, moderate, and severe impairment.

Symptomatic Psychiatric Assessment:

The objective of symptomatic diagnostic systems such as those in the DSM-IV is to classify behavioral disorders, provide decision rules for differential treatment, offer information regarding outcomes of disorders with and without treatment, and encourage systematic inquiry when differential treatment effectiveness is unknown (American Psychiatric Association, 1994; Taylor, 1983). Except in the case of general medicine and psychiatry, symptomatic diagnosis is rarely used in treatment planning. Although some diagnoses imply specific treatments, most do not.

The diagnostic criteria for major depressive disorder are: a depressed mood or newly developed loss of interest or pleasure in almost all activities for at least 2 weeks; changes in behavior that cannot be attributed to physical causes; no evidence of delusions or hallucinations; and behavior that is not a normal reaction to the death of a loved one. In addition, at least five of the following items must be present during this same 2-week period:

- Daily or near-daily occurrence of depressed mood or loss of pleasure

- Significant weight loss or gain (i.e., more than 5%)

- Problems in falling asleep, staying asleep, or sleeping too much

- Psychomotor agitation or retardation

- Fatigue

- Feelings of worthlessness or guilt

- Problems with concentration

- Recurrent thoughts of death, suicidal ideation, or an actual suicide attempt

At present, with the exception of dysthymia, no diagnostic age restriction exists regarding the onset of depression. Currently, the research data are equivocal with respect to the occurrence, characteristics, and need for a separate diagnostic category of late-onset depression (Koenig & Blazer, 1992).

Structured Psychiatric Interviews

Structured interviews are valuable due to the specific format of questioning and the empirical base established through clinical research. Such interviews allow the counselor to make differential diagnostic decisions early in the counseling process; consequently, the counselor can begin to tailor interventions to the identified behavioral disorder. The disadvantages of structured clinical interviews are the rigid style in which the questions are phrased, the potentially impersonal nature of the interview, the training required to learn to use the instrument correctly, and the length of the interview. Some of these impediments can be overcome through practice and training. Despite the apparent rigor of such interviews, considerable clinical judgment is still required to score a client's response.

The Schedule for Affective Disorders and Schizophrenia (SADS) is currently regarded as the "gold standard" in the field of structured psychiatric interviews (Endicott & Spitzer,

1978). It consists of two parts — current status and historical information — and contains more than 100 questions. The interviewer rates the answers to the questions by using a seven-point, Likert-type scale. Information gathered in Part 1 focuses on the multiple aspects of depression, including recent problems or difficulties, the client's reason(s) for seeking counseling, the time the difficulties began, and whether things are worse now than before. The information obtained allows the interviewer to determine the onset of the depressive disorder and to pinpoint whether the condition is chronic. It takes approximately 90 minutes to complete Part 1. Part 2 is completed if the diagnostic decision is not clear-cut and if a history of behavioral dysfunction is of interest. At the end of the interview, the client completes a Global Assessment Scale to rate the overall functioning over the past week.

The SADS is sensitive to detecting major depressive disorder in depressed and nondepressed older adults. It also contains questions about thought disturbance and alcohol use. A briefer version, SADS-Change Interview, can be used at repeated interviews to evaluate the change in diagnostic status and specific behavioral items. Although the SADS-Change Interview is the preferred SADS instrument for clinical practice, the original SADS is recommended as the clinical interview when working with older adults (Gallagher, 1986). However, data on SADS still need to be supplemented by medical information, mental status test results, and behavioral assessment findings.

Self-Reported Depression Scales

Numerous self-reported depression scales have been developed. The most frequently used and widely known scales will be briefly reviewed for their strengths and weaknesses with older adults. (Interested readers may consult other sources for comprehensive reviews of these measures; Gallagher & Thompson, 1983a; Kochansky, 1979; McNair, 1979). Although such instruments cannot be used for diagnosis, they do provide timely information regarding problem severity and do identify global behaviors that aid in the selection of specific target behaviors. These instruments can be used at each session or at the beginning and end of counseling to measure the outcome. As a result, self-reported depression scales are especially useful in nonresearch counseling settings.

The Zung Self-Rating Depression Scale (SDS) (Zung, 1965) is a widely used instrument with younger and middle-age adults. The psychometric properties of the instrument are acceptable with these age groups. However, the same results have not been obtained with older adults (McGarvey, Gallagher, Thompson, & Zelinski, 1982). The Zung SDS has been shown to be minimally discriminatory between depressed and nondepressed older adults. In addition, the Zung SDS has a heavy somatic bias that negatively affects older adults; that is, depression scores are inflated. As a result, the Zung SDS is not highly recommended for use with older adults.

Another widely used depression screening scale is the Beck Depression Inventory (BDI) (Beck, Ward, Mendelsohn, Mock, & Erbaugh, 1961). The BDI long form consists of 21 items that are rated using a four-point, Likert scale to measure intensity. A single numerical score is obtained by adding the individual ratings. Clinical convention holds that the following cutting scores be used: 0–9=normal, 10–15=mild, 16–19=mild to moderate, 20–29=moderate to severe, and 30–63=severe depression. The reliability of the BDI with older adults has been addressed by Gallagher and colleagues (Gallagher, Nies & Thompson, 1982; Gallagher, Breckenridge, Steinmetz, & Thompson, 1983). The results of this research, which used large samples of older adults, suggest that the BDI is sensitive and reliable in detecting self-reported depression in older adults. Test-retest and Chronbach's coefficient (a measure of internal consistency) are 0.90 and 0.91, respectively. When a BDI cutoff score of 17 was used, 91% of clients obtaining such scores were found to be independently diagnosed as experiencing major depression using the SADS. Prior work by Schwab and colleagues (Schwab, Bialow, Clemmons, Martin, & Holzer, 1967; Schwab, Bialow, & Holzer, 1967) as well as Nielsen and Williams (1980) with younger medical inpatients suggests that cutoff scores ranging from 1 to 13 be used on the BDI long form to detect depression. Few data are available regarding the use of the BDI with geriatric medical inpatients.

Potential problems with the BDI in older adults include readability, scaling, and somatic bias of the items. The BDI requires an eighth-grade education to understand the items. Furthermore, the role of somatic complaints in the diagnosis and assessment of depression raises concerns regarding the use of the BDI in older adults (Talbott, 1991). Dessonville and colleagues (1982) reported that it was difficult to interpret somatic items on the BDI for nondepressed adults older than 70 years of age who reported poor health. These results suggest that somatic items on the BDI should be replaced or that different self-report rating scales should be used (Rapp & Vrana, 1989).

The recently developed Geriatric Depression Scale (GDS) has attempted to address the issues of readability, scaling, and somatic bias (Yesavage et al., 1983). The GDS consists of 30 dichotomously scaled (yes/no) items addressing the verbal (cognitive), emotional, and motor aspects of depression. Scores range from 1 to 30, with higher scores indicating more severe depression. A cutoff score of 11 has been found to result in an 84% sensitivity and a 95% specificity regarding diagnosis of depression in community-dwelling older adults (Brink et al., 1982). Use of the GDS with medical inpatients and stroke patients has produced sensitivity and specificity rates ranging from 88%–92% and 64%–89%, respectively (Agrell & Dehlin, 1989). Preliminary evidence suggests that the GDS has a five-factor structure: (a) sad mood and pessimism, (b) loss of cognitive and physical energy, (c) positive or happy mood, (d) agitation and restlessness, and (e) social withdrawal (Sheik et al., 1991). Overall, the GDS is a user-friendly, highly reliable, and sensitive index of self-reported depression.

Behavioral Analysis:

The purpose of behavioral assessment is to identify the target (problem) and alternative behaviors, determine variables that influence the occurrence of maladaptive behavior, aid in the development of *prescriptive* interventions, and provide a baseline from which to evaluate treatment progress (Haynes, 1987; Nelson & Hayes, 1986).

Several guidelines are available for behavioral assessment. They can be neatly summarized under the acronym SORC — Stimuli, Organismic variables, Responses, and Consequences (Goldfried & Sprafkin, 1976). Moreover, these guidelines are helpful in forming behavioral counseling tactics.

Stimuli

The emphasis is placed on the assessment of functional (manipulable) relationships among biologic and environmental variables (Williamson, Waters, & Hawkins, 1986). Antecedents are events that precede the occurrence of behavior(s). They may be overt or covert and may occur across four domains: verbal/cognitive, visceral/emotional, motor, and physical/environmental. Such events function as discriminatory stimuli and "signal" (or set the occasion for) behavior. For example, the wandering behavior of a spouse with Alzheimer's disease residing in a nursing home may be the antecedent for the occurrence of the wife's private (covert) verbal response, "A good wife takes care of her husband at home," as well as avoiding future visits to the nursing home and experiencing feelings of dysphoria.

In contrast to theories of trait behavior, the behavioral model assumes a high degree of *situation specificity* and, correspondingly, a *low degree* of inference in the occurrence of behavior. The implication is that there are *multiple* idiosyncratic determinants for behavior. The assumption of *individualized* causal variables increases the importance of pre-intervention assessment. More important, historic interactions with the environment affect the *current* behavioral repertoire and its relationships with the current social environment (Hayes, 1989).

Organismic Variables

Physiologic systems and responses are considered organismic variables. Situational variables (antecedent conditions) outside the organism are monitored by receptors of vision, hearing, taste, smell, warmth, pressure, and pain. Internal events are monitored by interoceptors (within organs of the body) and proprioceptors (located within connective tissue and the inner ear). These events are then acted upon by higher integrative systems (e.g., central nervous system), resulting in changes in behavior at multiple levels of analysis. The integration of sensory information and output of the integrative system can be influenced by biologic variables or environmental events. A biologic example includes impaired memory due to neurofibrillary tangles associated with Alzheimer's disease. Changes in overt motor or emotional responses may be observed by enhancing relevant antecedent or consequent events (Hussian & Brown, 1987; Rodman, Gantz, Schneider, & Gallagher-Thompson, 1991).

Responses

Behavioral dysfunction can be expressed across four modes of responses: overt verbal, covert verbal (cognitive), overt motor, and physiologic. Emotional behavior may be expressed through overt verbal, motor, and physiologic modes. Modes of response may have low levels of response covariation. The degree of covariation depends on the person, the mode of response, and the disorder. Finally, many behaviors are interdependent. Table 9.3 offers an example of the multimodal pattern of depressed behavior.

In many cases, the modification of one behavior affects others in the *response class*, such as depression. For example, an increase in pleasant activities alters motor, emotional, and cognitive behavior. Finally, there are individual differences in the response topography of the behavioral disorder. For example, some persons may cry when depressed, whereas others may not cry at all but spend an inordinate amount of time sleeping. Behavioral disorders, such as depression, are the products of multiple biobehavioral causal pathways. Consistent with the focus on biobehavioral relationships is an emphasis on the behavioral *skills* of a client. It is assumed that the

	Table 9.3 ANALYSIS OF DEPRESSED BEHAVIOR	
Behavior	*Behavioral Deficits*	*Behavioral Excess*
Motor	Decreased social involvement Decreased self-care Decreased sexual behavior Decreased sleep; early awakening; waking during the night Minimal/slow motor behavior	Restlessness Agitation Increased sleep Suicide attempts
Verbal	Decreased communication Decreased positive statements about self, others, and the world	Increased complaints about money, job, family, neighbors, physical health, and guilt; talk of suicide
Emotional	Loss of sensitivity to pleasure	Reports of sadness, (anhedonia), emotionally "numb," boredom, failure, helplessness, hopelessness, worthlessness; crying; irritability
Physiologic	Decreased appetite; weight loss	Increased complaints of dizziness; fatigue; immunosuppression gastrointestinal problems, constipation, indigestion; chest pain, tachycardia; generalized aches and pains

client's behavioral repertoire defines the breadth and severity of the behavioral disorder.

Consequences

Consequences are the reinforcing or punishing events that maintain or increase the occurrence of behavior (positive and negative reinforcement) and suppress responses (punishment). From a traditional operant perspective, the consequences of behavior must be defined in terms of external environmental events. In such a model, antecedent and consequent events that control behavior ultimately lead to the external environment as the distal *and* proximal cause of the behavior. With complex human behavior, where verbal responses (cognitions) are important, it is often difficult to explain why behavioral patterns are observed in the absence of immediately obvious, contemporary environmental consequences. Consider the case of a caregiver with depression who continues to provide care despite increased feelings of dysphoria. Such behavior may be maintained by the avoidance of more aversive consequences, such as feelings of failure and disrespect. The avoidance of these events represents negative reinforcement and maintains the caregiving behavior. "Rule-following behavior" itself ("a good wife takes care of her husband at home") may also be the source of positive reinforcement that maintains complex human behavior over long periods (Lewin & Lundervold, 1990; Hayes, 1989; Skinner, 1969). Intermittent social reinforcement regarding caregiving serves to strengthen the rule-following behavior.

Observational Methods

Behavioral assessment aims to identify specific maladaptive behaviors, the contexts within which such behaviors occur, and the extent to which intervention affects change in behavior in the criterion setting. As such, direct observation and self-recording of behavior in the natural environment are indispensable parts of the assessment and counseling process. Structured clinical interviews and self-report screening instruments focus only on verbal reports of the severity of behavior and do not provide information regarding antecedent and consequent events controlling behavior. Such instruments provide an incomplete sample of behavior with no immediate or direct information regarding the *unique* circumstances and behavior of the client, which is needed to provide *prescriptive* counseling interventions.

Generally speaking, behavioral assessment of depression can be categorized according to ABC records, activity schedules, daily mood ratings, informant ratings, and direct observation of social interactions. ABC records are self-recorded descriptions of *antecedents*, *behaviors*, and *consequences* relevant to counseling for depression. Activity schedules are measures of the frequency and degree of enjoyment of pleasant events that a client has engaged in within a specified period. Daily mood ratings provide an index of how one's mood fluctuates during the day and are related to antecedents and consequences in the environment. Mood ratings are usually obtained four times a day, with ratings based on a nine-point scale. Informants can provide mood ratings as well as ratings of how often and how enjoyable activities are to a family member. Such ratings are valuable sources of information and should not be overlooked. Finally, direct observation of social interactions and engagement in activities can be conducted. Specially designed coding systems are used to assess dysphoria, attention, complaints, and other behaviors (Hopps et al., 1990).

BEHAVIORAL APPROACHES TO DEPRESSION

The first attempt to conduct a functional analysis of depression was performed by Skinner (1953). Skinner described depression as the weakening of behavior due to the interruption of established sequences of behavior that had been positively reinforced by the social environment. This theoretical analysis has been central to all subsequent behavioral theories of depression.

Behavioral therapies continued with the work of Ferster (1966), who provided more detail by suggesting an array of factors that could result in depressed behavior, including sudden environmental changes, punishment, aversive control, and changes in reinforcement contingencies (e.g., higher rates of response for lower rates of social reinforcement). Consistent with Skinner's views, Ferster suggested that slowing of motor (psychomotor retardation) and verbal behavior (thinking) was a function of the reduction in the performance of positively reinforced behavior.

Ferster also made an important observation regarding restricted social interactions and the resulting patterns of behavior. Persons with depression are limited in the array of environmental contexts within which they interact, thus making them vulnerable to change. Their behavior becomes passive rather than interactive with the environment. As Hanley and Baike (1984) pointed out, these two observations appear to be especially relevant for older adults whose social contexts are limited and who become the passive recipients of care through lack of adequate finances, social skills, or environmental control. The social environment of the person provides well-intended but counterproductive attention and sympathy, which serve to strengthen and maintain depressed behavior. However, these interactions eventually become aversive and result in withdrawal of social reinforcement, thus exacerbating depression.

Costello (1972) suggested that depression was due to a lack of effectiveness on the part of the reinforcer rather than the loss of reinforcers *per se*. Such a loss can be attributed to biological or environmental variables and is especially relevant to older adults. Deterioration in physical and sensory functions will decrease the salience of reinforcers.

Reinforcement can be contingent or noncontingent on behavior. Noncontingent reinforcement of behavior results in idiosyncratic and maladaptive patterns across all modes of response. Verbal behavior may be especially sensitive to the effects of noncontingent reinforcement or punishment (Hayes, Kohlenberg, & Melacon, 1989; Hineline & Wachisen, 1989; Poppen, 1989).

In summary, analysts of clinical behavior have demonstrated that depression and reinforcement are related phenomena. Depression is defined as a response class comprised of an array of behaviors that vary, and reinforcement is defined as positive social and physical environmental interactions. Depressed behavior is a function of low rates of contingent reinforcement, lack of effectiveness on the part of the reinforcer, and increased rates of aversive consequences. This state of affairs may be a result of: few available positive reinforcers or an increased number of aversive consequences in the person's social environment, social-skills deficits that limit access to positive interactions with the environment or aid in coping with stressful circumstances, maladaptive behavioral patterns that limit the opportunity and access to and/or potency of positive events, and the diminished potency of positive reinforcers and/or the heightened salience of aversive consequences.

Behavioral Counseling Interventions:

Behavioral counseling interventions are typically designed to be short-term (usually 4–15 sessions) and are applied in a structured format. As part of the therapeutic contract, a limited number of sessions are determined in the initial session and used to help the client and counselor define and accept counseling goals. Goals are established through a collaborative process between the counselor and client and are renegotiated as needed. The behavioral rationale for the onset, maintenance, and improvement in mood is thoroughly discussed within the first few sessions. Finally, the tactics of the counseling intervention are determined, ideally based on an individualized behavioral analysis of the unique circumstances of each case. This refers to the specific intervention used with a client. In general, these interventions fall into three categories: (a) a change in the physical environment (e.g., relocation); (b) simple skill acquisition (i.e., one behavior is targeted for change); and (c) complex skill acquisition (i.e., multiple behavioral targets).

Behavioral counseling approaches that use complex skill acquisition models target a variety of behaviors for change, including: participation in pleasant activities, social skills, and self-statements. Complex models are generally referred to as *cognitive-behavioral or cognitive interventions*. In either case, the inclusion of verbal behavior (self-statements, beliefs) as a target of intervention or behavioral change is consistent with

a behavioral analytic account of depressed behavior, especially with regard to the role of rule-governed behavior (Hayes,
1989; Lewin & Lundervold, 1990; Poppen, 1989; Salzinger,
1992; Skinner, 1969). Cognitive *theory* places greater emphasis
on beliefs that may lead to depression (rule-governed behavior) and hypothetical cognitive structures as the central and
causative factors of depression. Changes in overt and emotional behavior are viewed as merely "symptoms" (Beck &
Weishaar, 1989). Yet, cognitive *therapy* is more problem-ori-
ented and behavioral with regard to self-recording of behavior, increasing pleasant events, and teaching accurate discrimination of behavior-environment and behavior-behavior
relationships.

Group Outpatient Counseling:

Simple Skill Acquisition

Lovett and Gallagher (1988) conducted a large-scale clinical
trial that evaluated activity schedules (pleasant events) and
problem-solving counseling interventions for older adults
with depression. Participants were primarily older adult caregivers of family members with heterogeneous disabilities.
Approximately 50% met the SADS criteria for major or minor
depressive episodes. Ten weekly group sessions lasting 2
hours were conducted. Compared with a waiting-list control
group, caregivers who participated in each counseling intervention reported decreased depression and increased morale.

The "increasing life satisfaction" (activity schedules) counseling intervention was modeled after that of Lewinsohn,
Munoz, Youngren, and Zeiss (1986). Caregivers were taught to
monitor their mood and pleasant events, identify pleasant
events in which they wished to engage, establish step-by-step
goals for increasing pleasant events, and evaluate their progress
in achieving these goals. In the problem-solving condition,
caregivers were taught a systematic procedure for specifying
problems, generating possible solutions, evaluating advantages and disadvantages of solutions, selecting the best solution, and implementing a plan of action based on the solution.

Individual problems of the caregivers were used to teach the skills. Problem-solving counseling produced results similar to those obtained by increasing pleasant events.

Complex Skill Acquisition

Few studies have been conducted in a group format using the complex skill acquisition model. Steuer and associates (1984) compared cognitive-behavioral and psychodynamic group counseling in a mixed group of older adults (55 years or older) with depression. After 46 sessions, lower BDI scores were obtained for older adults receiving cognitive-behavioral counseling compared with the comparison group. Based on BDI scores, 15% of the patients receiving the cognitive-behavioral counseling were free of depression at the end of the intervention period. Two more patients were classified as mildly depressed. No follow-up results were reported.

Individual Outpatient Counseling:

Simple Skill Acquisition

Teri and Uomoto (1991) successfully used activity schedules with older adults with coexisting dementia and depression. Caregivers were taught to monitor the disabled family member's mood and the frequency and duration of pleasant events. Next, pleasant events were identified using a structured screening instrument, and the caregiver was taught to increase the frequency and duration of events infrequently engaged in by the family member. Significant increases in the mood and number of activities engaged in by the disabled family member resulted from the intervention. Also of great importance is the finding that the caregivers, who were moderately depressed and met DSM-IV criteria for major depression prior to intervention, benefited from rehabilitation of the disabled family member. After intervention, caregivers were free of depression.

Complex Skill Acquisition

Gallagher and colleagues conducted a number of studies

evaluating individual cognitive, behavioral, and interpersonal-psychodynamic counseling approaches (Gallagher-Thompson et al., 1990; Gallagher & Thompson, 1982; Gallagher & Thompson, 1983b; Thompson, Gallagher, & Breckenridge, 1987). In this series of studies using three approaches, brief individual counseling was conducted over 16 to 20 sessions within a 12-week period. Cognitive counseling focused on the primary role of dysfunctional beliefs as the cause of depression and consisted of a variety of behavioral interventions to make the client more aware of the relationship among thoughts, feelings, and overt behavior. Behavioral counseling targeted increases in pleasant events and social skills. Finally, interpersonal-psychodynamic counseling aimed at uncovering "deep" intrapsychic conflicts (Horowitz & Kaltreider, 1979).

Based on the BDI and Hamilton Depression Scale, no statistically significant differences in outcomes were reported with the various interventions (Hamilton, 1967). Changes in GDS scores showed more improvement for older adults receiving behavioral counseling. Long-term follow-up (2 years) of 91 older adults indicated that 70% of the participants were free of depression after therapy.

Group Inpatient Counseling:

Simple Skill Acquisition

Hussian and Lawrence (1981) used problem solving and prompting and social reinforcement of engagement in activities with nursing home residents with BDI scores in the moderate-to-severe range. Problem-solving training was based on standard methods and was conducted by trained recreation therapy assistants. Assistants also provided verbal prompts and praise for engagement in activities. The interventions were compared with a waiting-list control group and an attention control group. Five sessions per week for 2 weeks were conducted. Outcome measures were based on BDI scores and a self-rating of depression measuring frequency, intensity, and duration of depression.

When comparing preintervention and postintervention BDI scores with self-rating scale scores, a difference in self-rating scale scores was obtained. A 2-week follow-up revealed significant changes in the BDI and self-rated depression scale scores when the combined problem-solving and activities intervention was compared. At 3 months, significant differences among treatments emerged only after both measures were combined. Based on BDI cutting scores, 4 residents who received problem-solving or social reinforcement for engagement in activities experienced mild depression or none at all.

Complex Skill Acquisition

One study using a complex model of behavioral counseling has been conducted with older adults in an inpatient setting. Brand and Clingempeel (1992) used group behavioral counseling to increase pleasant events and social skills; their approach was modeled after that of Gallagher and Thompson (1981). A total of 53 older adults participated in 16 sessions of group behavioral counseling held 4 times a week for 2 weeks. All group members received medication. Behavioral group counseling was compared with standard hospital treatment, which consisted of pharmacotherapy, occupational therapy, and individual sessions with treatment team members. All participants were older than 60 years of age and diagnosed with major depressive disorder. The levels of therapeutic medication did not differ.

Outcome measures included the BDI, the Hamilton Rating Scale for Depression, and the Depression Scale of the Nurses' Observation Scale for Inpatient Evaluation (Hoenigfeld, 1966). Traditional statistical analysis of group averages resulted in no differences among groups on any of the measures. The authors then conducted clinical evaluations of change scores on individual cases. They used clinical cutoff scores to determine clinically significant change for each patient. This analysis indicated that a greater number of patients who received behavioral group counseling were not depressed after treatment when compared with patients who underwent standard hospital treatment. With the Hamilton Rating Scale, 44% of the patients who underwent behavioral group counseling were "in remission," compared with 15% of patients who underwent standard intervention. Using the BDI, 27% were within the normal range. Twenty-six percent of the patients in the behavioral group were in the "normal" range on the BDI and "in remission" on the Hamilton Rating Scale. A total of 2% of the patients who underwent standard intervention achieved this outcome.

SUMMARY

The results of individual or group behavioral counseling validate its use based on research with heterogeneous samples of older adults with major depressive disorder. Compared with a waiting-list control group, behavioral counseling interventions produced significantly greater improvements in self-reported and counselor-rated depression. Additional research using individual counseling formats has been conducted in outpatient settings. Further, a limited number of studies have been conducted with geriatric inpatients, and both simple and complex behavioral counseling interventions have been used with equal effectiveness. Simple models have focused on problem solving and improving pleasant events, whereas complex models have relied on altering dysfunctional rules and improving social skills. No studies have been conducted to determine which method is more efficacious for which clients.

None of the studies discussed conducted a behavioral analysis of depressed behavior for the individual case. However, "package treatment" approaches were used, and all patients were treated the same regardless of their current behavioral skills, deficits, and circumstances. The results of Brand and Clingempeel (1992) highlight this issue. The package treatment used by these clinical counselors was most effective with patients who *already* had a high base-rate performance of these skills. These results indicate the need for a behavioral analysis of the individual case and prescriptive intervention (McNight, Nelson, Hayes, & Jarrett, 1984). Such an approach avoids the "myth of homogeneity" inherent in symptomatic diagnosis while maximizing effective counseling outcomes (Biglan & Dow, 1981).

REFERENCES

Agrell, B., & Dehlin, O. (1989). Comparison of six depression rating scales in geriatric stroke patients. *Stroke, 22,* 1190–1194.

Aldwin, C. M., Spiro, A. III, Levenson, M. R., & Brosse, R. (1989). Longitudinal findings from the study of normal aging, I: Does mental health change with age? *Psychology and Aging, 4,* 295–306.

American Psychiatric Association. (1994). *Diagnostic and statistical manual of mental disorders.* (4th ed.) Washington, DC: Author.

Beck, A. T., Ward, C., Mendelsohn, M., Mock, J., & Erbaugh, J. (1961). An inventory for measuring depression. *Archives of General Psychiatry, 4,* 561–571.

Beck, A. T., & Weishaar, M. E. (1989). Cognitive therapy. In R. J. Corsini & D. Wedding (Eds.), *Current psychotherapies* (4th ed., pp. 285–322). Itasca, IL: FE Peacock.

Biglan, A., & Dow, M. G. (1981). Toward a 'second generation' model of depression treatment: A problem-specific approach. In L. P. Rehm (Ed.), *Behavior therapy for depression: Present status and future directions.* New York: Academic Press.

Blazer, D., Hughes, D. C., & George, L. K. (1987). The epidemiology of depression in an elderly community population. *Gerontologist, 27,* 281–287.

Blazer, D., & Williams, C. D. (1980). Epidemiology of dysphoria and depression in an elderly population. *American Journal of Psychiatry, 137,* 439–444.

Bourgeois, M. S. (1990). Enhancing conversational skills in patients with Alzheimer's disease using a prosthetic memory aid. *Journal of Applied Behavior Analysis, 23,* 29–42.

Brand, E., & Clingempeel, W. G. (1992). Group behavioral therapy with depressed geriatric inpatients: An assessment of incremental efficacy. *Behavioral Therapy, 23,* 475–482.

Brink, T. L., Yesavage, J. A., Owen, L., Heersema, P. H., Adey, M., & Rose, T. (1982). Screening tests for geriatric depression. *Clinical Gerontology, 1,* 37–43.

Cohen, D., & Eisdorfer, C. (1988). Depression in family members caring for a relative with Alzheimer's disease. *Journal of the American Geriatrics Society, 36,* 885–889.

Costello, C. G. (1972). Depression: Loss of reinforcers or reinforcer effectiveness? *Behavioral Research and Therapy, 3,* 240-247.

Dessonville, C., Gallagher, D., Thompson, L. W., Finnell, K., & Lewinsohn, P. M. (1982). Relation of age and health status of depressive symptoms in normal and depressed older adults. *Essence, 5,* 99–117.

Endicott, J., & Spitzer, R. L. (1978). A diagnostic interview for affective disorders and schizophrenia. *Archives of General Psychiatry, 35,* 837–844.

Ferster, C. B. (1966). Animal behavior and mental illness. *Psychological Record, 16,* 345–356.

Folstein, M. F., Folstein, S., & McHugh, B. (1975). Mini-mental state exam: A practical method of grading the cognitive state of patients for the clinician. *Journal of Psychiatric Research, 12,* 189–198.

Gallagher, D. (1986). Assessment of depression by interview methods and psychiatric rating scales. In L. Poon (Ed.), *Handbook for clinical memory assessment of older adults* (pp. 202-212). Washington, DC: American Psychiatric Press.

Gallagher, D., Breckenridge, J. N., Steinmetz, J., & Thompson, L. W. (1983). The Beck Depression Inventory and research diagnostic criteria: Congruence in an older adult population. *Journal of Consulting and Clinical Psychology, 51,* 945–946.

Gallagher, D., Nies, G., & Thompson, L. W. (1982). Reliability of the Beck Depression Inventory with older adults. *Journal of Consulting and Clinical Psychology, 50,* 152–153.

Gallagher, D., & Thompson, L. W. (1981). *Depression in the elderly: A behavioral treatment manual.* Los Angeles: University of Southern California Press.

Gallagher, D., & Thompson, L. W. (1982). Differential effectiveness of psychotherapies for the treatment of major depressive disorder in older adults. *Psychotherapy: Theory, Research, and Practice, 19,* 482–490.

Gallagher, D., & Thompson, L. W. (1983a). Depression. In P. M. Lewinsohn & L. Teri (Eds.), *Clinical geropsychology* (pp. 1-37). New York: Pergamon Press.

Gallagher, D., & Thompson, L. W. (1983b). Effectiveness of psychotherapy for both endogenous and nonendogenous depression in older adult outpatients. *Journal of Gerontology, 38,* 707–712.

Gallagher-Thompson, D., Hanley-Peterson, P., & Thompson, L. W. (1990). Maintenance of gains following brief psychotherapy for depression. *Journal of Consulting and Clinical Psychology, 58,* 371–374.

Goldfried, M. R., & Sprafkin, J. N. (1976). Behavioral personality assessment. In J. T. Spence, R. C. Carson, & J. W. Thibaut (Eds.), *Behavioral approaches to therapy* (pp. 295–321). Morristown, NJ: General Learning Press.

Hamilton, M. (1967). Development of a rating scale for primary depression. *British Journal of Social and Clinical Psychology, 7,* 278–296.

Hanley, I., & Baike, E. (1984). Understanding and treating depression in the elderly. In I. Hanley & J. Hodge (Eds.), *Psychological approaches to the care of the elderly* (pp. 213-236). New York: Methuen.

Hayes, S. C. (1989). *Rule-governed behavior: Cognition, contingencies, and instructional control.* New York: Plenum Press.

Hayes, S. C., Kohlenberg, B. S., & Melacon, S. M. (1989). Avoiding and altering rule-control as a strategy of clinical intervention. In S. C. Hayes (Ed.), *Rule-governed behavior: Cognition, contingencies, and instructional control* (pp. 358-388). New York: Plenum Press.

Haynes, S. N. (1987). Behavioral assessment of adults. In M. Hersen & A. Bellack (Eds.), *Handbook of psychological assessment* (pp. 369-401). New York: Pergamon Press.

Hendricks, J., & Hendricks, C. D. (1977). *Aging in mass society*. Cambridge, MA: Winthrop.

Hineline, P. N., & Wachisen, B. A. (1989). Correlated hypothesizing and the distinction between contingency-shaped and rule-governed behavior. In S. C. Hayes (Ed.), *Rule-governed behavior: Cognition, contingencies, and instructional control* (pp. 221-268). New York: Plenum Press.

Hoenigfeld, G. (1966). NOSIE: Nurse Observation Scale for Inpatient Evaluation. In W. Guy (Ed.), *ECDEU assessment manual for psychopharmacology*. Rockville, MD: National Institute of Mental Health.

Hopps, H., et al. (1990). *Living in Family Environmen.s (LIFE) coding system*. Eugene, OR: Oregon Research Institute.

Horowitz, M., & Kaltreider, N. (1979). Brief therapy of the stress response syndrome. *Psychiatric Clinics of North America, 2*, 365–377.

Hussian, R. A., & Brown, D. C. (1987). Use of two-dimensional grid patterns to limit hazardous ambulation in demented patients. *Journal of Gerontology, 42*, 558–560.

Hussian, R. A., & Lawrence, P. S. (1981). Social reinforcement of activity and problem-solving training in the treatment of depressed institutionalized elderly patients. *Cognitive Therapy and Research, 5*, 57–69.

Incalzi, R. A., Gemma, A., Capparella, O., Muzzolon, R., Antico, L., & Carboni, P. U. (1991). Effects of hospitalization on affective status of elderly patients. *International Psychogeriatrics, 3*, 67–74.

Jarvik, L. A., & Perl, M. (1981). Overview of physiologic dysfunction related to psychiatric problems in the elderly. In A. J. Levenson & R. C. W. Hall (Eds.), *Neuropsychiatric manifestations of physical disease in the elderly*. New York: Raven Press.

Kochansky, G. E. (1979). Psychiatric rating scales for assessing psychopathology in the elderly: A critical review. In A. Raskin & L. A. Jarvik (Eds.), *Psychiatric symptoms and cognitive loss in the elderly* (pp. 125-156). Washington, DC: Hemisphere.

Koenig, H. G., & Blazer, D. G. (1992). Mood disorders and suicide. In J. E. Birren, et al. (Eds.), *Handbook of mental health and aging* (pp. 380-409). New York: Academic Press.

Koenig, H. G., Meador, K. G., Cohen, H. J., & Blazer, D. G. (1988a). Depression in elderly hospitalized patients with medical illness. *Archives of Internal Medicine, 148,* 1929–1936.

Koenig, H. G., Meador, K. G., Cohen, H. J., & Blazer, D. G. (1988b). Self-rated depression scales and screening for major depression in older hospitalized patients with medical illness. *Journal of the American Geriatrics Society, 36,* 699–706.

LaRue, A., D'Elia, L. F., Clark, E. O., Spar, J. E., & Jarvik, L. A. (1986). Clinical tests of memory in dementia, depression, and healthy aging. *Journal of Psychology and Aging, 6,* 69–77.

Lewin, L. M., & Lundervold, D. A. (1990). Behavioral analysis of separation-individuation in the spouse of an Alzheimer's disease patient. *Gerontologist, 30,* 703–705.

Lewinsohn, P. M., Munoz, R. A., Youngren, M. A., & Zeiss, A. M. (1986). *Control your depression.* Englewood Cliffs, NJ: Prentice-Hall.

Lovett, S., & Gallagher, D. (1988). Psychoeducational interventions for family caregivers: Preliminary efficacy data. *Behavioral Therapy, 19,* 321–330.

McGarvey, B., Gallagher, D., Thompson, L. W., & Zelinski, E. (1982). Reliability and factor structure of the Zung Self-Rating Depression Scale in three groups. *Essence, 5,* 141–151.

McNair, D. M. (1979). Self-rating scales for assessing psychopathology in the elderly. In A. Raskin & L. A. Jarvik (Eds.), *Psychiatric symptoms and cognitive loss in the elderly* (pp. 157-167). Washington, DC: Hemisphere.

McNight, D. L., Nelson, R. O., Hayes, S. C., & Jarrett, R. B. (1984). Importance of treating individually assessed response classes in the amelioration of depression. *Behavioral Therapy, 15,* 315–335.

Nelson, R. O., & Hayes, S. C. (1986). *Conceptual foundations of behavioral assessment.* New York: Guilford Press.

Newman, J. P. (1989). Aging and depression. *Psychology and Aging, 4,* 150–165.

Nielsen, A. C., & Williams, T. A. (1980). Depression in ambulatory medical inpatients: Prevalence in self-report questionnaire and recognition by nonpsychiatric physicians. *Archives of General Psychiatry, 37,* 99–104.

Parmalee, P. A., Katz, I. R., & Lawton, M. P. (1992). Depression and mortality among institutionalized aged. *Journal of Gerontology, 47,* 3–10.

Poppen, R. L. (1989). Some clinical implications of rule-governed behavior. In S. C. Hayes (Ed.), *Rule-governed behavior: Cognition, contingencies, and instructional control* (pp. 325-358). New York: Plenum Press.

Rapp, S., & Vrana, S. (1989). Substituting nonsomatic for somatic symptoms in the diagnosis of depression in elderly male medical patients. *American Journal of Psychiatry, 146,* 1197–1200.

Rodman, J. L., Gantz, F. E., Schneider, J., & Gallagher-Thompson, D. (1991). Short-term endogenous depression using cognitive-behavior therapy and pharmacotherapy. *Clinical Gerontology, 10,* 81–85.

Rovner, B. W., et al. (1990). The prevalence and management of dementia and other psychiatric disorders in nursing homes. *International Psychogeriatrics, 2,* 13–24.

Ruegg, R. G., Zisook, S., & Neal, N. R. (1988). Depression in the aged. *Psychiatric Clinics of North America, 11,* 83-99.

Salzinger, K. (1992). Cognitive therapy: A misunderstanding of B. F. Skinner. *Journal of Behavior Therapy and Experimental Psychiatry, 23,* 3–8.

Schulz, R., Visintainer, P., & Williamson, G. M. (1990). Psychiatric and physical morbidity effects of caregiving. *Journal of Gerontology, 45,* 181–191.

Schwab, J. J., Bialow, M. R., Clemmons, R., Martin, P., & Holzer, C. (1967). The Beck Depression Inventory with medical inpatients. *ACTA Psychiatrica Scandinavica, 43,* 255–266.

Schwab, J. J., Bialow, M. R., & Holzer, C. E. (1967). A comparison of two rating scales for depression. *Journal of Clinical Psychology, 23,* 94–96.

Sheik, J. I., et al. (1991). Proposed factor structure of the Geriatric Depression Scale. *International Psychogeriatrics, 3,* 23–28.

Skinner, B. F. (1953). *Science and human behavior.* New York: Free Press.

Skinner, B. F. (1969). *Contingencies of reinforcement.* New York: Appleton Century Crofts.

Steuer, J., et al. (1984). Cognitive behavioral and psychodynamic group therapy in the treatment of geriatric depression. *Journal of Consulting and Clinical Psychology, 54,* 180–189.

Talbott, M. M. (1991). Age bias in the Beck Depression Inventory: A proposed modification for use with older women. *Clinical Gerontology, 9,* 23–26.

Taylor, C. B. (1983). DSM-III and behavioral assessment. *Behavioral Assessment, 5,* 5–14.

Teri, L., & Uomoto, J. M. (1991). Reducing excess disability in dementia patients: Training caregivers to manage patient depression. *Clinical Gerontologist, 10,* 49–64.

Teri, L., & Wagner, A. (1992). Alzheimer's disease and depression. *Journal of Consulting and Clinical Psychology, 60,* 379–391.

Thompson, L. W., Gallagher, D., & Breckenridge, J. (1987). Comparative effectiveness of psychotherapies for depressed elders. *Journal of Consulting and Clinical Psychology, 55,* 385–390.

Weissmann, M. M., & Myers, J. K. (1979). Depression in the elderly: Research directions in psychopathology, epidemiology, and treatment. *Journal of Geriatric Psychiatry, 13,* 187–210.

Williamson, D. A., Waters, W. F., & Hawkins, M. F. (1986). Physiologic variables. In R. O. Nelson & S. C. Hayes (Eds.), *Conceptual foundations of behavioral assessment* (pp. 297-327). New York: Guilford Press.

Yesavage, J., et al. (1983). Development and validation of a geriatric depression screening scale: A preliminary report. *Journal of Psychiatric Research, 17,* 37–49.

Zarit, S. H. (1980). *Aging and mental disorders: Psychological approaches to assessment and treatment.* New York: Free Press.

Zung, W. W. K. (1965). A self-rating scale for depression. *Archives of General Psychiatry, 12,* 63–70.

10

The Management and Resolution of Dependency in the Depressed Client

John A. Birtchnell, MD, FRC Psych., DPM, Dip. Psychother.,
AFBPsS

Dr. Birtchnell is Honorary Senior Lecturer at the Institute of
Psychiatry, and Honorary Consultant Psychiatrist at the Maudsley
Hospital, London, England.

KEY POINTS

- A strong relationship exists between pathologic dependency and depression. Only pathologic dependence is linked to depression; therefore, distinguishing between normal and patho-logic dependence is essential.

- Pathologic dependence is characterized by an excessive need to be loved; a general feeling of inadequacy and incompetence; a persistent need for guidance, reassurance, and approval; a tendency to take rather than to give; an inclination to relate to others in a humble and apologetic manner; and maturational deficiencies.

- The object of counseling is to correct maturational deficiencies, which requires a rerun of the client's childhood. The counselor takes on the role of the alternative parent.

- The dependent personality has its complementary counterpart: the dominant personality or the *powerful other*; dominant persons need to be needed and prefer to play the dominant role in relationships. If a client has a relationship with a dominant partner, it is often advantageous to involve the partner in counseling sessions.

- A review of therapeutic goals and methods for counseling dependent, depressed clients is presented.

THEORETICAL BACKGROUND: DEPENDENCE

It is unwise to present an account of the management of the depressed client who is dependent without first considering what dependence is and what relationship it bears to the state of being depressed. In general, people assume that dependence is more common in women than in men. This may be related to the increased vulnerability that women have to developing depression.

WHAT IS DEPENDENCE?

Distinguishing between normal and pathologic dependence is essential (Birtchnell, 1991a), for only pathologic dependence is linked with depression. Birtchnell (1984, 1988) described pathologically dependent people as childish. Parens and Saul (1971) emphasized that dependence is a normal feature of childhood. As maturity is reached, it becomes less evident. Mahler (1963), however, correctly drew attention to Freud's assertion that a life-long, albeit diminishing, emotional dependence upon the mother is a universal truth of human existence and that at times it is quite appropriate for adults to be dependent.

Dependence is a complex phenomenon that cannot be defined simply (Birtchnell, 1984). When pathologic, it has the following characteristics: an excessive need to be loved, cherished, and made a fuss of; a general feeling of inadequacy and incompetence; a persistent need for guidance, reassurance, and approval; a tendency to take rather than to give; and an inclination to relate to others in a humble and apologetic manner from a lowly and submissive position.

One way to view pathologic dependence is as a failure of maturity, and any therapeutic approach to it should involve the facilitation of further maturation. Essentially, pathologically dependent people have failed: (a) to adequately separate initially from their mothers and subsequently from their families of origin, (b) to establish a well-defined and secure identity, (c) to acquire an approving and nonjudgmental internal-ized parent and in consequence an appropriate sense of self-worth, and (d) to consider themselves to be worthy of joining the world of adults (on equal footing with other adults).

HOW IS PATHOLOGIC DEPENDENCE CREATED AND MAINTAINED?

It seems likely that dependent people have failed to attain an adequate level of maturity because they have not been encour-aged or permitted to do so by their dominant maternal figure and other members of their families of origin. If dependent people remain in contact with their mothers or families, the family members will continue to play a part in maintaining the dependence. In terms of transactional analysis, as described by Berne (1975), dependent people have well-developed child ego states but deficient adult and parent states. They can therefore only relate to others as would children to their parents. They need to induce other adults to adopt a parental attitude toward them. Millon (1981) described how dependent persons search for a "single, all-powerful, magical helper" on whom they can project a parental image and in whom they can place trust. Once such an attachment has been formed, little opportunity for change remains and the dependent position is maintained.

We should not forget that there also exists a complementary personality type who needs to be needed and who prefers to play the dominant role in relationships (Birtchnell, 1987). In transactional-analysis terms, people who have such a person-ality type have a well-developed parent ego state but deficient adult and child states. They seek out people who will become dependent upon them and apply pressure on those with whom they relate to coerce them into assuming a more subordinate role. People with a dominant personality find dependent people attractive and dependent people, in turn, are attracted to them. If their need to be dominant is compelling, they may draw out latent dependent behavior even in relatively nondependent people. This type of personality is not uncommon among doctors, nurses, psychiatrists, counselors, and even psychotherapists. These features can be a serious handicap in the management of dependence.

When treating dependent clients, counselors must consider their own personalities and attitudes toward clients, the extent of the clients' continued involvement with members of their families of origin and the effect that such involvement is having on their clients, the personalities of other key figures in the dependent clients' lives, how capable they are of modifying their style of relating to the clients, and the attitude and behavior of other professionals involved in the clients' care. Whatever good work may be done in counseling sessions can effectively be undone by parents and significant others with whom the dependent clients live and have contact.

THE RELATIONSHIP BETWEEN DEPENDENCE AND DEPRESSION

Bemporad (1980) observed that pathogenic dependency may be the one characteristic of depressed people that has been unanimously emphasized in the psychiatric literature. Fast (1967) wrote of the intense feeling of total dependence on others that one sees in persons prone to depression. Bibring (1953) referred to the "orally dependent type" who thrives on "oral narcissistic supplies," the lack of which he considered to be the most frequent type of predisposition to depression. Gaylin (1968), in the preface to a collection of psychoanalytic papers on depression, wrote, ". . .there is hardly a theory of depression that does not in some way emphasize orality." Rado (1968) referred to depression as "a great despairing cry for love," and Fenichel (1968) described the depressed person as a "love addict" who is in a perpetual state of greediness. Millon (1981) observed that dependent people's need for affection and assurance that they will not be abandoned may become so persistent as to exasperate and alienate those upon whom they lean most heavily. This only serves to increase their neediness. When others inevitably reject them, a cycle of decompensation begins. Overt expressions of self-criticism, self-blame, and self-condemnation come fore and ultimately progress to frank depressive symptoms.

Research Evidence:

Bullock and colleagues (1972) observed an intensification of dependent behavior by women when they were depressed. These women wanted to be told what to do and have decisions made for them. The dependency took on a demanding quality, which was often a source of irritation and confusion to their husbands, who fluctuated between being overprotective and doubting their need for help. It is of some interest that approximately half of the 57 items on the Dependency Scale of the MMPI refer to aspects of depression, but clients who score high on the depressive items also score high on the remaining items (Birtchnell & Kennard, 1983). Hirschfeld and colleagues (1977) developed a relatively depression-free measure of dependence and demonstrated that depressed clients have significantly higher scores than normal persons (Hirschfeld et al., 1983a). Following recovery, their dependence scores dropped but still tended to remain significantly higher than those of never-depressed persons (Hirschfeld et al., 1983b).

The Two Main Components of Dependence:

In a more recent review (Birtchnell, 1991b), nine characteristics of depression were listed and compared with published characteristics of the dependent personality disorder. Evidence suggests that dependence may have two major components, which could be called *closeness* and *lowerness*. Birtchnell (1993) proposed that these components correspond with two types of depression, one concerned with loss of close involvement and the other with loss of status. They have connections types of depression, one concerned with loss of close involvement and the other with loss of status. They have connections with what Beck (1983) called *deprivation depression* and *defeat depression*. An empirical study (Birtchnell, Falkowski, & Steffert, 1992) confirmed that depressed people do have both high closeness and high lowerness scores. This is significant for counseling in that it helps to determine which component of dependence the depression is associated with and to direct attention toward alleviating that component.

Self-Esteem — The Vital Link:

Beck (1967) observed that the precipitants of depression are often situations that would be expected to lower self-esteem. Hirschfeld and associates (1976) proposed that a drop in self-esteem marks the onset of clinical depression and considered that depression-prone people have a chronically low level of self-esteem. McCrainie (1971) maintained that depressive affect is a direct response to lowered self-esteem, and Rado (1968) considered that persons who are predisposed to depression are wholly reliant and dependent on other people for maintaining their self-esteem. Chodoff (1972) defined dependence as the degree to which a person's self-esteem is maintained more or less exclusively by the approval and support of other persons or their surrogates, and Nemiah (1975), explaining the onset of neurotic depression, described how people who are abnormally dependent on others find themselves in difficulty when faced with situations that lower their self-esteem. He pointed out that normal people who find their self-esteem assaulted and diminished by various situations and events restore their emotional equilibrium by putting their setbacks into proper perspective, balancing a failure in one direction with success in another. Dependent people lack the inner resources that would sustain them in times of adversity. Storr (1983) proposed that normal children acquire a kind of built-in self-esteem from early positive relationships with their mothers.

THE POWERFUL OTHER

Fast (1967) described the belief common to many depressed people that they are helplessly dependent on others (originally their mothers) who are responsible for their present misery and the only possible source of rescue from it. They see their situation as one centrally involving rejection by the powerful other and themselves as helplessly dependent on the other to reinstate them as good, acceptable, loved, and a part of a meaningful life. Bemporad (1980) referred to the dominant other as the person who gives meaning to the depressed person's life. Depressed people have ceased to respond to their own psychic interior and derive pleasure only from gaining the approval of the dominant other. They have a fear of what Bemporad called "autonomous gratification," seeking to please themselves by becoming actively involved in rewarding activities that give them personal satisfaction. Instead, they enter into a "bargain relationship" in which they deny themselves personal pleasures in return for nurturance from the dominant other.

DEPENDENCE AND SUICIDAL INCLINATION

Both research and clinical evidence (Birtchnell, 1981, 1983) indicate that dependent persons commonly attempt to commit suicide. Tabachnick (1961) argued that people who attempt suicide are often more dependent than normal in a rather infantile manner. Schwartz, Flinn, and Slawson (1974) described the suicidal character type as that form of the generally dependent character type in which the suicidal threat or attempt is the specific device by which assistance is coerced from others. The suicidal impulse appears strongest when a relationship to a significant other has broken down or is in danger of breaking down. Draper (1976) suggested that the ever-present "pain-in-living" of the suicidal adult may represent a reexperiencing of the inconsolable pain of the helpless infant, wittingly or unwittingly deserted by the mother in whom he or she has put all his or her affection, libidinal hopes, and pleasures. Draper referred to the mother as "the ONE." The pain returns when the adult later encounters loss of the ONE in a selected transference object. "It is not difficult to see," he wrote, "the link between the loss of a vitally important person who has become draped (no matter what his actual sexual identity) with the powerful mantle of the first loving figure, the ONE."

THERAPEUTIC AIMS AND METHODS

Opinions vary on the importance of counseling in the treatment of depression. Bemporad (1980) expressed the view that it is the most effective treatment of mild depression, and Arieti (1980) maintained that, although the presenting symptoms of severe depression may be removed by nonpsychotherapeutic measures, the client remains vulnerable to further episodes without the adjunct of counseling. Because the treatment of depression needs to address a number of issues, the present review is artificial in that it is restricted to considerations of dependence, either as a manifestation of the depression itself or as a component of vulnerability to it.

COUNSELING

The Initial Contact:

Counselors' initial responses to dependent clients will be determined by each client's circumstances and emotional state. During a period of crisis, when a critical relationship has been broken or is under strain, pain-in-living will be intense (Draper, 1976). Clients undergoing such periods will be inclined to regress and to cling desperately, and their counselors will have little option but to offer themselves as attachment objects. This may even require physically holding the client. A desperately clinging client can arouse strong anxiety in a counselor; acknowledgment of this should deter him or her from taking evasive action. For awhile, the counselor will remain the client's reason for living. The counselor should be respectful of this and avoid any action that may be interpreted as rejection.

Even at less critical times, dependent clients' persistent needs for closeness can feel like an intrusion into the counselors' personal space, and counselors may respond by being intolerant and hostile. Keeping these feelings in check, however, is a necessary requirement for successful counseling. Millon (1981) observed that dependent people tend to seek assistance whenever they can and are all too receptive to being involved in treatment. Dependent clients are comforted by the strength and authority of counselors and feel assured that the counselors will provide them with the kindness and helpfulness they crave. Bemporad (1980) pointed to the seductiveness of dependent clients, whose praise and flattery can be a source of narcissistic gratification to unwary counselors. Dependent clients' care-eliciting maneuvers can, at times, evoke an overprotective and nurturing response. It is easy to swing too far in the direction of making promises that are impossible to keep.

The Counseling Plan:

The object of counseling is to correct, belatedly, the maturational deficiencies that were enumerated under the definition of dependence. This requires a kind of rerun of the client's childhood. The counselor inescapably takes on the role of alternative parent.

Although the transient intense dependence of depressed clients is fairly readily resolvable, correction of the persistent dependence trait of depression-prone clients may require months or even years. Management of the separate components of dependence will be considered in sequence.

Love:

Because a number of researchers have emphasized the hunger for love in dependent clients, particularly when they are depressed, it is reasonable to consider whether, and to what extent, counselors should offer dependent clients the love they crave. It might be permissible, in moments of extreme crisis, to offer a direct and unambiguous show of love. In one such situation, Dublin (1985) wrote, "I will love the hell out of him." Many dependent clients certainly recall that they did not experience their mother's love as unrestrained and freely given. Instead, it had a forced and unreal quality. The conventional clinical detachment of the counselor may be perceived as frustratingly similar. Therefore, it seems likely that progress will be limited unless the counselor actually comes to like the client and, within the safe confines of the counseling session and when appropriate, can make a show of genuinely caring feelings.

Separation:

Throughout the course of counseling, two distinct, although interrelated, separation issues must be considered. The first is clients' separation from their mothers and families of origin; the second is separation from the counselors. To some extent, clients' attachment to the counselors, albeit temporary, makes attempts at separation from mothers and families easier. Clients' must be helped to be more aware of their mothers' devices for keeping them. These may center on the issue of the mother's need of the client, with the mother inclined to play upon his or her sense of obligation and loyalty. In this case, the client swings from pangs of guilt over his or her wish to break free to outbursts of anger because the mother will not let him or her go.

Clients may still be living with their mothers or be in regular contact by visit, letter, or telephone, so they should be encouraged to try various degrees of confrontation, which may be rehearsed or reported on during counseling sessions. Some advantage may exist in inviting a client's mother to some sessions; there, each may come to appreciate more clearly what it feels like to be the other. The mother may resort to an all-or-nothing declaration — either the client stays or goes completely. The prospect of a complete break can fill the client with such anxiety that he or she will abandon all attempts to increase separation. Alternatively, with the assured support of the counselor, he or she may choose and adhere to a complete break. Such a drastic measure is a common resolution of the conflict. If the mother is dead or out of contact, the process of more complete separation must be worked through entirely on a subjective level.

Separation from the counselor can be no less difficult, and it may occur on the "micro" or the "macro" level. Dependent clients may be so concerned that they will lose their counselors that they may try to extend sessions by introducing problematic material toward the end or may simply feel unable to leave. They may try to telephone their counselors between sessions to ask for extra appointments or make suicidal threats or gestures. Counselors must make clear to clients how much time they can offer and try not to deviate from that. They must assure clients that they do care about them but will care neither more nor less in response to any manipulative maneuvers. At the "macro" level, clients will try to extend the course of counseling beyond its optimal length. Counselors must recognize that they may be the recipient of a powerful transference and must therefore gently ease their clients away, allowing them the option of further contacts over a protracted period. It is always preferable for clients to take responsibility for the final break.

The Establishment of a More Definite and Secure Identity:

The establishment of a secure identity runs hand in hand with the process of becoming more separate. Staying close to the mother involves sharing her identity, just as staying close to the family involves sharing the family identity. Mahler (1961) put the twin processes of becoming separated and becoming a separate person together into the single term *separation-individuation.* Bowen's (1978) differentiation of self from the family of origin carries the implication of breaking away and starting anew as a different person. He referred to the "emotional stuck-togetherness or fusion" in the nuclear family and of the need for the client to attain a state of emotional objectivity from his or her parents. This is equivalent to what others have referred to as autonomy. Ideal adult relationships develop between two autonomous persons. A person who has not attained the state of individuation, differentiation, objectivity, or autonomy can only relate to another by fusion.

An important feature of the counseling of dependent clients is helping them develop the capacity to gradually build up identities that are recognizably their own. They should be encouraged to seek out that small nucleus of self that they do have and progressively add to it. To this end, they should repeatedly be invited to express their opinions and to make choices. They should be offered opportunities to discover their likes and dislikes, to do the things they think would give them pleasure, and to fully experience the pleasure they derive from doing such things.

What makes this exercise difficult for them is the disloyalty they come to experience either to their parents or to some other emotionally important person. Arieti (1980) wrote, "Step by step we must clarify to the client that he does not know how to live for himself. He has never listened to himself or been inclined to assert himself, but cared only about obtaining the approval, affection, love, admiration, or care of the dominant other." Counselors must appreciate the fact that clients have, up to this point, lived only for the praise of others. They find it hard to conceive of an existence in which their actions are motivated by their own sense of personal satisfaction. The transition from living to please another to living in response to inner needs may be accompanied by feelings of isolation, inertia, or futility. Having abandoned one lifestyle, they may experience a time lag before they can establish a new one. They may readily slip into a kind of pseudoautonomy in which they create the impression of self-motivation in order to gain their counselors' approval.

The Acquisition of Inner Resources:

It is one thing to establish a sense of self and quite another to develop an appropriate evaluation of that self. Dependent people tend to be completely at the mercy of the judgments of those around them. They find it difficult to tell whether what they say or do is good or bad. They must therefore extend their efforts toward determining what they like or dislike, including themselves and the things that they do.

The gestalt principle of urging dependent clients to accept and to own unashamedly everything that is part of themselves, particularly their bodies, will have a powerful, reinforcing effect. Most dependent persons believe themselves to be incapable of doing anything well. It is necessary for counselors to point to clients' positive qualities and achievements and persuade them to acknowledge their obvious worth.

Counseling sessions usually reveal that one of the client's parents had a persistently disparaging attitude toward him or her and was grudging in praise or approval. It is important that he or she be made aware of this and helped to understand why this parent needed to behave in this way. It is impossible to totally expunge a bad internalized parent, but the client should be helped to view the parent's behavior more objectively and be less influenced by the parent's former view of him or her.

During the course of counseling, the counselor will inevitably come to assume a parental image, and his or her more positive view of the client will hopefully counteract the actual parent's negative view.

Enabling Clients to Accept Themselves as Adults:

Parents should make clear to their children the demarca-

tion, within the family, between the older and younger generation and the behavior that is appropriate to each. As children
grow older, they should be permitted gradually to assume a
more adult status and eventually arrive at the level of their
parents. For dependent persons, this gradual progression to
an adult status has been interrupted; they have become fixated
at the child level. The situation is usually complicated by the
fact that they have become involved in one or more relationships in which they play out the role of the child to a dominant
other, who reciprocally plays parent to them.

During the initial stages of counseling, it will be difficult to
be anything other than relatively dominant to a client who is
behaving in such a conspicuously submissive manner. Such a
client knows no other way of relating, and his or her belief that
it is the counselor's job to solve his or her problems and make
him or her better will not be easily dispelled. Bemporad (1980)
argued that regression in counseling is definitely to be avoided,
that the use of the psychoanalytic couch is not advisable, and
that giving in to clients' demands may provide symptomatic
relief but will not affect his underlying patterns of thought.
Eventually, he warned, the client will demand more and more.
This is not necessarily so.

When a client is in a depleted state, a limited period of
indulgence, even to the point of regression, may be necessary
to restore his or her emotional reserves. The client will not
necessarily demand more and more. The ultimate objective is,
of course, to progress gradually toward a relationship in
which the counselor and the client interact on an adult-to-
adult basis. The strategies referred to in the previous two
sections for establishing a strong identity, increasing autonomy,
and improving self-esteem will obviously contribute to this.
At the same time, the counselor must increasingly decline to
respond to the client's appeals for guidance and reassurance
and instead treat him or her as though he or she were a
competent and responsible adult.

Clients may carry with them from childhood a deep-seated
fear of growing up and a conviction that they have no right to
behave as adults. This emotional distortion is maintained by a

powerful superego and a disapproving and punitive internalized parent. More superficial treatment approaches will fail, and premature attempts to coerce clients toward more adult behavior will be blocked unless this fundamental issue is confronted. A degree of controlled catharsis may be necessary, during which clients will alternate between self-punishing guilt and vengeful rage toward the suppressive parent. Such emotion will be directed, through the transference, onto the counselor. Additionally, the counselor will present himself or herself as an alternative, more benign parent, who will ease the client's emergence into adulthood.

In terms of transactional analysis, clients have come to adopt dependent scripts, which they are able to maintain by entering into relationships with others who are willing to play the complementary dominant role. They rely heavily upon their child ego state; their adult and parent ego states need to be built up. Dusay (1986) observed that strengthening weaker ego states is like exercising an underdeveloped muscle. Clients need a great deal of practice and encouragement from others who must be prepared to abandon their own excessively parental behavior toward the clients.

MANAGEMENT OF DEPENDENT SUICIDAL CLIENTS

Dependent people experience acute anxiety and intense psychic pain whenever their relationship to a supportive other person is broken or weakened. The pain may be such that it drives them to actual suicide; more often, they only attempt or threaten it. Initially, the suicidal attempt or threat will evoke an increased caring response in the supportive other, but subsequently it may come to have the opposite effect. When hospitalized or in counseling, dependent clients may react suicidally to fears that the hospital staff or counselor does not really care about them. In turn, the caregivers may respond by showing increased concern or by being more protective or restraining. This response makes clients feel frightened by their lack of trust in them and, as a result, they become helpless and even more needful of them. Frequently, such a situation sets up a vicious circle in which repeated suicide attempts are followed by increasing concern and restraint. Schwartz and colleagues (1974) emphasized the need to break this vicious circle by encouraging clients to progressively take more responsibility for themselves. They likened the situation to that of the overprotective parent who prevents the child from acquiring a confidence in coping with everyday hazards by not exposing him or her to such hazards.

INVOLVEMENT OF SIGNIFICANT OTHERS IN COUNSELING

Outside of counseling, dependent clients may be involved in a number of relationships that keep them in dependent attitudes and behavior. One of these may be the continuation into adult life of the relationship with their mothers, or other parental figures, from which their dependency grew. There may be at least one other relationship in which they have totally or partially reproduced this original relationship. For his or her own personal reasons, the dominant partner in such a relationship may prefer to remain dominant and resist the dependent client's attempts to be more assertive or self-reliant. Not infrequently, two dependent people form a relationship and compete with each other for the dependent position. In all these situations, there are advantages to drawing the significant other into the counseling sessions.

The continuing relationship with the original parent, being of the longest duration, is usually the most difficult to change. The parent has an investment in keeping the client weak and needy and is not likely to see any advantage to allowing him or her to break free. Sessions that include the parent may, however, make it easier for the client — in the presence of the counselor — to stand up to and pull away from the parent. The counselor, by being supportive of the parent, may be able to help him or her accept this.

Counseling sessions with the dominant other are more likely to succeed. The dominant other has two principal fears: one, that if he or she loses control, the relationship will get out of hand; the other, that if he or she relaxes his or her dominant facade, he or she may find it necessary to reveal his or her own vulnerability. The therapeutic objective should be to allow the client to discover that the dependent partner is capable of acting responsibly without posing too great a threat to his own position in the relationship and to reassure the client that it is not too disastrous to expose his or her own weaknesses to the dependent partner, who may in fact sometimes welcome the opportunity to be caring and sympathetic toward him or her.

Relationships between two dependent persons are notoriously unstable. Each is afraid to allow the other to become too separate or too autonomous, and so each thwarts the other's efforts in these directions. Each feels unloved and yet resents the other's receiving any love. Such relationships sometimes assume sadomasochistic characteristics, because the partners take turns to hurt or be hurt: when one is up, the other is down. Suicide attempts by either partner are common. For one partner, through counseling, to become less dependent, spells disaster for the other. Ideally, therefore, each should be in counseling, but this should be supplemented by conjoint counseling.

The essential strategy for attempting to modify the relationship with a significant other is preventing excessive anxiety in either member of the relationship. When anxiety is aroused by the possibility of change, each member will dig in and adhere even more strongly to his or her present role. Progress can be made by suggesting a series of small shifts, in which one partner will agree to give way in one direction at the same time and to the same extent as the other agrees to give way in a complementary direction (Birtchnell, 1986).

REFERENCES

Arieti, S. (1980). Psychotherapy of severe depression. In S. Arieti & J. Bemporad (Eds.), *Severe and mild depression: The psychotherapeutic approach*. London: Tavistock Publications.

Beck, A. T. (1967). *Depression: Clinical, experimental, and theoretical aspects*. New York: Harper & Row.

Beck, A. T. (1983). Cognitive therapy of depression: New perspectives. In P. J. Clayton & J. E. Barrett (Eds.), *Treatment of depression: Old controversies and new approaches*. Philadelphia, PA: University of Pennsylvania.

Bemporad, J. (1980). Psychotherapy of mild depression. In S. Arieti & J. Bemporad (Eds.), *Severe and mild depression: The psychotherapeutic approach*. London: Tavistock Publications.

Berne, E. (1975). *What do you say after you say hello?* London: Corgi.

Bibring, E. (1953). The mechanism of depression. In P. Greenacre (Ed.), *Affective disorders: Psychoanalytic contributions to their study*. New York: International Universities Press.

Birtchnell, J. (1981). Some familial and clinical characteristics of female, suicidal, psychiatric patients. *British Journal of Psychiatry, 138*, 381-390.

Birtchnell, J. (1983). Psychotherapeutic considerations in the management of the suicidal patient. *American Journal of Psychotherapy, 37*, 24-36.

Birtchnell, J. (1984). Dependence and its relationship to depression. *British Journal of Medical Psychology, 57*, 215-225.

Birtchnell, J. (1986). The imperfect attainment of intimacy: A key concept in marital therapy. *Journal of Family Therapy, 8*, 153.

Birtchnell, J. (1987). Attachment-detachment, directiveness-receptiveness: A system for classifying interpersonal attitudes and behaviour. *British Journal of Medical Psychology, 60*, 17-27.

Birtchnell, J. (1988). Towards a definition of dependence. *British Journal of Medical Psychology, 61*, 111-123.

Birtchnell, J. (1991a). Redefining dependence: A reply to Cadbury's critique. *British Journal of Medical Psychology, 64,* 253-261.

Birtchnell, J. (1991b). The measurement of dependence by questionnaire. *Journal of Personality Disorders, 5,* 281-295.

Birtchnell, J. (1993). *How humans relate: A new interpersonal theory.* Westport, CT: Praeger.

Birtchnell, J., Falkowski, J., & Steffert, B. (1992). The negative relating of depressed patients. *Journal of Affective Disorders, 24,* 165-176.

Birtchnell, J., & Kennard, J. (1983). What does the MMPI dependency scale really measure? *Journal of Clinical Psychology, 39,* 532-543.

Bowen, M. (1978). *Family therapy in clinical practice.* London: Aronson.

Bullock, R. C., et al. (1972). The weeping wife: Marital relations of depressed women. *Journal of Marriage and the Family, 34,* 488-495.

Chodoff, P. (1972). The depressive personality: A critical review. *Archives of General Psychiatry, 27,* 666-673.

Draper, E. (1976). A developmental theory of suicide. *Comprehensive Psychiatry, 17,* 63-80.

Dublin, J. E. (1985). The terrorized patient as brutalized person. In E. M. Stern (Ed.), *Psychotherapy and the terrorized patient.* New York: Hawthorn Press.

Dusay, J. M. (1986). Transactional analysis. In I. L. Kutash & A. Wolf (Eds.), *Psychotherapist's casebook.* London: Jossey-Bass.

Fast, I. (1967). Some relationships of infantile self-boundary development to depression. *International Journal of Psychoanalysis, 48,* 259-266.

Fenichel, O. (1968). Depression and mania. In W. Gaylin (Ed.), *The meaning of despair.* New York: Science House.

Gaylin, W. (1968). The meaning of despair. In W. Gaylin (Ed.), *The meaning of despair.* New York: Science House.

Hirschfeld, R. M. A., et al. (1976). Dependency-self-esteem-clinical depression. *Journal of the American Academy of Psychoanalysis, 4,* 373-388.

Hirschfeld, R. M. A., et al. (1977). A measure of interpersonal dependency. *Journal of Personality Assessment, 41,* 610-618.

Hirschfeld, R. M. A., et al. (1983a). Assessing personality: Effects of the depressive state on trait measurement. *American Journal of Psychiatry, 140,* 695-699.

Hirschfeld, R. M. A., et al. (1983b). Personality and depression: Empirical findings. *Archives of General Psychiatry, 40,* 993-998.

Mahler, M. S., (1961). On sadness and grief in infancy and childhood. *Psychoanalytic Study of the Child, 16,* 332.

Mahler, M. S. (1963). Thoughts about development and individuation. *Psychoanalytic Study of the Child, 18,* 307.

McCrainie, E. J. (1971). Depression, anxiety, and hostility. *Psychiatric Quarterly, 45,* 117-133.

Millon, T. (1981). *Disorders of personality, DSM-III: Axis II.* New York: Wiley & Sons.

Nemiah, J. C. (1975). Depressive neurosis. In A. M. Freedman, H. I. Kaplan, & B. J. Sadock (Eds.), *Comprehensive textbook of psychiatry 101* (Vol. 1). Baltimore: Williams & Wilkins.

Parens, H., & Saul, L. J. (1971). *Dependence in man: A psychoanalytic study.* New York: International Universities Press.

Rado, S. (1968). The problem of melancholia. In W. Gaylin (Ed.), *The meaning of despair.* New York: Science House.

Schwartz, D. A., Flinn, D. E., & Slawson, P. F. (1974). Treatment of the suicidal character. *American Journal of Psychotherapy, 28,* 194-207.

Storr, A. (1983). A psychotherapist looks at depression. *British Journal of Psychiatry, 143,* 431-435.

Tabachnick, N. (1961). Interpersonal relations in suicidal attempts. *Archives of General Psychiatry, 4,* 16-21.

11

Treatment of Depression and the Restoration of Work Capacity

Jim Mintz, PhD, Lois I. Mintz, PhD, Mary Jane Robertson, MS, Robert P. Liberman, MD, and Shirley M. Glynn, PhD

For authors' affiliations, see page 223

KEY POINTS

- Among workers with depressive symptoms, functional work impairment is quite common.

- Even mild work difficulties or complaints may be early warning signs of depression in some persons. Such problems include diminished productivity, chronic lateness, feeling ashamed of one's work, sudden loss of job interest, absenteeism, interpersonal tensions, and other work difficulties.

- Such early subjective complaints of affective work impairment deserve careful evaluation, particularly in a person who is vulnerable to depressive episodes. Early detection can lead to early intervention.

- In many cases, it may not be possible to determine whether difficulties at work are a result or a cause of depression. Often, clients are caught in a vicious downward cycle in which work-related problems and depressive symptoms exacerbate each other.

- Psychotherapy appears to be associated with somewhat slower rates of work recovery than treatment with antidepressant medications.

- An effective medication can be expected to reduce depressive symptoms in as few as 4–6 weeks. However, full restoration of work capacity may require 4–6 months.

INTRODUCTION

Depressive disorders are among the most prevalent psychiatric conditions, and impairment in occupational or major-role functioning is a common complication. Depressive symptoms are frequent concomitants of many medical disorders, so the issue of depression and its effects on functioning is highly relevant to primary care health providers. An overemphasis on symptom remission has resulted in the unfortunate neglect of improved occupational and social functioning as a critical treatment goal, both in clinical practice and research.

This chapter first discusses the reciprocal influences of depression and work functioning. Then, we present some issues and difficulties inherent in measuring work impairment in depressed clients. We describe the results of a large-scale, multiproject study of the specific impact that treatments of depression have on occupational functioning.

DEPRESSION AND FUNCTIONAL IMPAIRMENT

Persons with major depressive disorder, as well as those with dysthymic disorder and depressive disorder not otherwise specified (NOS), are high users of medical services and are as functionally impaired as patients with severe chronic medical disorders (Depression Guideline Panel, 1993).

Mintz, Mintz, Arruda, and Hwang (1992) analyzed data from eight major studies of treatment of depression. They found that more than half (55%) of depressed patients met research criteria for work impairment at the time they entered treatment. Although there was some variability across the eight studies, on the average, nearly 11% of patients (range, 3%–20%) were unemployed and another 44% (range, 33%–69%) were classified as impaired workers (Mintz et al., 1992). According to epidemiologic data, patients with depression report more disability days than the general population (rates per 90-day interval: major depression, 11 days; dysthymia, 3 days; depression NOS, 4–6 days; general population, 2 days; Broadhead, Blazer, George, & Tse, 1990).

Based on results from the Medical Outcomes Study, Stewart and colleagues (1989) found that the presence of depressive symptoms was associated with a degree of impairment in functioning at work, home, or school; this impairment was comparable to, or even worse than, that associated with eight major chronic medical conditions, even when a clinical diagnosis of a depressive disorder was not present. Indeed, the degree of functional impairment associated with depressive symptoms was second only to that associated with advanced coronary artery disease. They declared that depression "is perhaps more like chronic medical conditions in terms of morbidity than has previously been appreciated" (Stewart et al., 1989).

Thus, the impact of depression on occupational productivity is an issue of profound societal importance. Data from the Epidemiologic Catchment Area (ECA) study (Weissman, Bruce, Leaf, Florio, & Holzer, 1991) indicate that depression is more prevalent in persons younger than 65 years of age — in essence, active members of the work force. A recent, widely publicized study by Greenberg, Stiglin, Finkelstein, and Berndt (1993) placed the total cost of affective disorder in terms of lost time and diminished productivity at more than $40 billion annually. Another estimate of the direct workplace cost of depression nationally, in terms of lost time at work, was more than 172 million days annually, based on 3%–5% 6-month prevalence rates for major depression alone (Dew, Bromet, Schulberg, Parkinson, & Curtis, 1991). Even if this estimate is somewhat high (recent data from the ECA study [Weissman et al., 1991] indicate the lifetime prevalence of major depression is 2.6% for men and 7% for women across all age groups), the cost is obviously considerable.

The direction of influence is not always easy to determine. In many cases, it may not be possible to determine whether difficulties at work are a result or a cause of depression. Often, patients are caught in a vicious downward cycle in which work-related problems and depressive symptoms exacerbate each other. Weissman and colleagues (1991) pointed out that men and women who have been unemployed for at least 6 months in the past 5 years are "more than three times as likely as others to have experienced a major depressive episode in the past year." They also noted that "it is difficult to interpret the causal direction in these relationships. They can suggest both that men and women with a history of affective disorders have greater difficulty obtaining and maintaining employment and that unemployed people are at greater risk of depressive episodes because they lack the sense of accomplishment, social bonds, time structure, and financial security provided by employment."

Evidence exists to suggest that job loss and fear of job loss can have dire psychological and psychiatric consequences (Hagen, 1983) and that reemployment has salutary effects on mental health (Caplan, Vinokur, Price, & van Ryn, 1989). Conversely, it is easy to see that symptoms of depression (such as frequent weeping; profound sadness or irritability; fatigue; lack of energy; loss of interest; slowing of thought, speech, and movement; agitation; somatic complaints, including headaches, or a more serious preoccupation with health) might well interfere with the capacity to work effectively.

DEPRESSIVE SYMPTOMS RELATED TO WORK IMPAIRMENT

Surprisingly enough, data that link specific depressive symptoms to work performance are quite sparse. Most studies have simply demonstrated a general link between the presence of depressive symptoms and functional incapacity. In fact, Anthony and Jansen (1984) cited several sources to bolster their contention that "there appear to be no symptoms or symptom patterns that are routinely related to individual work performance." The studies to which Anthony and Jansen refer relate primarily to the degree to which symptom severity during acute episodes predicts later work outcomes.

Liberman and colleagues (Liberman, 1989; Massel et al., 1990) concurrently evaluated work performance and symptoms in more than 600 clients with mental disorders. The data suggest that the conclusion of Anthony and Jansen (1984) is probably somewhat overstated and that there are significant, albeit modest, relationships between the severity of psychiatric symptoms and concurrently measured work output or productivity. Across all diagnostic groups, so-called negative symptoms appeared to be most strongly related to work dysfunction. (Glynn and associates [1992] also found negative symptoms to be the strongest correlates of work incapacity in a sample of schizophrenic patients.) Among depressed clients, motor retardation or slowing is probably the most crucial determinant of impaired productivity (Liberman, 1989).

TOOLS FOR ASSESSING WORK IMPAIRMENT

Extensive batteries for assessing work performance among clients with serious mental illness are used in vocational rehabilitation settings (e.g., the assessment battery developed by Cook and co-workers [1992]). However, psychiatric researchers in the areas of treatment and epidemiology have tended to rely on brief rating scales. This may be partly due to the fact that "functional limitations caused by depressive disorder are considered secondary to it, rather than part of its definition" (Wells et al., 1989).

Most scales for measuring work impairment rely heavily on self-reported data, raising the concern that even items relating to objective behaviors (such as absenteeism) can be subject to distortion through the lens of affective disturbance. After all, self-criticism, negativism, and pessimism are defining characteristics of depression. The value of actual measures of work performance is obvious; however, it would undoubtedly be a challenge to obtain such measures in both clinical and research contexts. An approach that has not been widely used outside the rehabilitation arena is evaluation with structured tasks or standardized work samples. This methodology, which is more widely used in vocational assessment than clinical research, has the appeal of standardization, replicability, and ease of quantification. However, its applicability across a range of abilities, jobs, work settings, and client populations is not clear (Cook et al., 1992).

Depression rating scales usually assess a variety of symptoms that may relate to work impairment, such as feelings of failure or lack of energy. However, none of the widely used scales specifically links particular symptoms with impairment at work. For example, the Beck Depression Inventory (Beck, Ward, Mendelson, Mock, & Erbaugh, 1961), a client self-report form, and the Hamilton Depression Rating Scale (Hamilton, 1960), designed to be completed by a clinician, are two of the most widely used research instruments for quantifying the severity of depressive symptoms. Each has only one item in which the word "work" even appears. On the Beck instrument (Table 11.1), the item confines itself to the concept of extra "effort" or "push" needed to "do anything." The Hamilton scale (Table 11.2) is somewhat more differentiated, alluding to increasingly severe levels of feelings of incapacity or inefficiency, the need to push to work, lack of interest and satisfaction, indecisiveness, clearly decreased efficiency, and lost time. On both scales, the inability to work in any regard receives the maximum score.

Table 11.1
WORK ITEM FROM THE
BECK DEPRESSION INVENTORY

0 = I can work about as well as before
1 = It takes an extra effort to get started at doing something
2 = I have to push myself very hard to do anything
3 = I cannot do any work at all

Table 11.2
WORK ITEM FROM THE HAMILTON
DEPRESSION RATING SCALE

---

0 = No difficulty
1 = Thoughts and feelings of incapacity, fatigue, or weakness related to activities
2 = Loss of interest in activity
3 = Decrease in actual time spent/decrease in productivity
4 = Stopped working because of present illness

Source: Beck, A. T., Ward, C. H., Mendelson, M., Mock, J., & Erbaugh, J. (1961).
An inventory for measuring depression. *Archives of General Psychiatry, 4,* 561–
571.

Functional impairment is assessed by the Rand 36-Item
Short-Form Health Survey (version 1.0), an instrument for
epidemiologic research referenced in the Medical Outcomes
Study (Wells et al., 1989) with three "yes/no" questions (Table
11.3) (Ware & Sherbourne, 1992). Although this simple assess-

---

Table 11.3
WORK ITEMS FROM THE RAND
36-ITEM SHORT-FORM HEALTH SURVEY

During the past 4 weeks, have you had any of the following problems with your work or other regular daily activities as a result of
any emotional problems (such as feeling depressed or anxious)?

Decreases in the amount of time
you spent on work or other activities .... Yes   No

Accomplished less than you would like .... Yes   No

Did not do work or other activities
as carefully as usual.. Yes   No

Source: Ware, J. E., & Sherbourne, C. D. (1992). The MOS 36-item short-
form health survey (SF-36), I: Conceptual framework and item selection.
Medical Care, 30, 473–483. Reprinted with permission from Lippincott-
Raven Publishers.

ment is rather nonspecific (both in terms of the functional and psychiatric domains involved), it does capture the core issues of diminished time, productivity, and quality of work. Moreover, it would be easy to incorporate into routine clinical assessment and screening.

In treatment-outcome research, the most commonly used instrument for assessing work adjustment has been the Social Adjustment Scale (SAS) (Schooler, Hogarty, & Weissman, 1979; Weissman & Bothwell, 1976; Weissman & Paykel, 1974), which has a section specifically devoted to assessment of work-role performance. We have reported that the 6 SAS work-role items (Table 11.4) fall broadly into two categories (Mintz et al., 1992). Three of the items evaluate behaviors (absenteeism, performance adequacy, and interpersonal conflict) and might be termed measures of *functional impairment*. Three other items evaluate subjective emotional states (distress, feelings of shame, and loss of interest) and thus might be termed *measures of affective impairment*. Norms published by Weissman, Prusoff, Thompson, Harding, and Myers (1978) from community samples of working men and women indicate that most workers report very good work adjustments. On the full 6-item SAS scale, the average score for more than 200 employed community residents of both genders was 1.3 (the scale ranges from 1 to 5), with a standard deviation of 0.3. Thus, a mean SAS work-role score as low as 2 is more than 2 standard deviations above the mean and would clearly place a client in the lowest 2%–8% of average working people in the community. Average scores of 3 or higher across the 6 items in Table 11.4 are virtually never seen in well-adjusted workers, and therefore are indicative of significant impairment.

Classifying Work Impairment:

In general, no accepted standard has been established for determining exactly when a depressed client should be classified as "impaired" in work function or for quantifying the degree of impairment. In 1992, we published the first major analyses of the effects of treatments of depression on functional work impairment (Mintz et al., 1992). The impetus for this project was a comprehensive review of the recent scientific literature on the effects of well-defined psychiatric treatments on outcomes in the workplace. The review of more than 4,000 research articles revealed that restoration of work capacity was a neglected topic in the psychiatric treatment literature, particularly in the case of affective disorders (Mintz, Mintz, & Phipps, 1992). We subsequently compiled data on work outcomes from 10 major studies of treatment for depression and analyzed them to determine the effects of treatment on work, to assess whether symptoms mediate work outcome, and to identify prognostic factors associated with work resto-

---

Table 11.4
WORK ITEMS FROM THE
SOCIAL ADJUSTMENT SCALE (SAS)

Functional Items

Time lost from work
1 = None
2 = 1 day
3 = Half the time
4 = More than half the time
5 = No days worked

Performance adequacy
1 = No impairment
2 = Adequate but some impairment
3 = Moderate impairment or did not work well about half the time
4 = Marked impairment or worked poorly most of the time
5 = Extreme impairment or worked poorly all the time

Friction/Avoidance
1 = No friction and smooth relationships
2 = Some mild friction but no avoidance
3 = Some friction and/or minimizes some contacts
4 = Moderate friction and/or minimizes many contacts
5 = Extreme friction or avoids/avoided by others

Table 11.4
WORK ITEMS FROM THE
SOCIAL ADJUSTMENT SCALE (SAS)
(CONTINUED)

Affective Items

Feelings of adequacy
1 = Almost always feels adequate or able to handle things, or never ashamed of work
2 = Usually or often feels adequate or able to handle things, or ashamed of work once or twice
3 = Sometimes feels adequate or able to handle things, or ashamed of work half the time
4 = Rarely feels adequate or able to handle things, or ashamed of work most of the time
5 = Almost never feels adequate or able to handle things, or ashamed of work all the time

Distress at work
1 = Not at all distressed
2 = A little distressed
3 = Moderately distressed or distressed half the time
4 = Very distressed or distressed most of the time
5 = Extremely distressed or distressed all the time

Interest in work
1 = Very interested
2 = Somewhat interested
3 = Neutral or not interested half the time
4 = Somewhat uninterested or not interested most of the time
5 = Very uninterested or not interested all the time

Sources: Schooler, N., Hogarty, G., & Weissman, M. (1979). Social Adjustment Scale II. In W. A. Hargreaves, C. C. Attkisson, & J. E. Sorenson (Eds.), *Resource materials for community mental health program evaluators* (Publication [ADM] 79328, pp. 290-203). Rockville, MD: U.S. Department of Health, Education, and Welfare; Weissman, M. M., & Bothwell, S. (1976). Assessment of social adjustment by patient self-report. *Archives of General Psychiatry, 31*, 37–42; Weissman, M. M., & Paykel, E. S. (1974). *The depressed woman: A study of social relationships.* Chicago, IL: University of Chicago Press.

ration. The 10 collaborating projects were controlled treatment studies performed under the supervision of many of the field's most prominent investigators (Clark & Fawcett, 1989; Davidson, Giller, Zisook, & Overall, 1988; Elkin et al., 1989; Fawcett et al., 1987; Frank et al., 1990; Frank, Kupfer, & Perel, 1989; Giller, Bialos, Riddle, & Waldo, 1988; Glick et al., 1985; Jarrett, Rush, Khatami, & Roffwarg, 1990; Murphy, Simons, Wetzel, & Lustman, 1984; Prusoff & Weissman, 1981; Quitkin et al., 1989; Rehm, Kaslow, & Rabin, 1987; Spencer et al., 1988; Stewart et al., 1988).

Clients were excluded from the project database if they were not in the active workforce (e.g., a housewife), were functioning adequately at the beginning of treatment, did not comply with treatment, or were missing crucial data (e.g., posttreatment assessment of either symptom or work outcome). A total of more than 800 depressed clients were included in the final analyses. Whenever possible, a consistent definition of symptom remission using conventionally accepted cutoff scores was applied to all studies. The most common measure was the Hamilton Depression Rating Scale.

Depressed clients were classified as *functionally impaired* (Table 11.5) at work if they reported significant absenteeism (missing half the scheduled work time or more); diminished productivity (at least moderate impairment or inadequate productivity at least half the scheduled time); significant interpersonal problems (many arguments or interpersonal conflicts with co-workers or supervisors, moderate friction, or avoidance of social contact); poor overall functioning (an average score of 2 or more on the 3 functional SAS items); or unemployment (the SAS role item includes a code for unemployed that is distinct from housewife or student roles). Occasionally, relevant ancillary data, such as a significant-life-events form (indicating the client had been fired), were available.

A measure of *affective work impairment* was also developed (Table 11.6). This latter measure was computed by averaging ratings of subjective adequacy (feelings of inadequacy, shame, or not being able to handle things at work); distress (feeling

---

Table 11.5
SAS-BASED CRITERIA FOR
FUNCTIONAL WORK IMPAIRMENT

Patients were operationally defined as functionally work impaired if they met any one of the following five criteria:

- *Absenteeism*: a score of 3 or more on the SAS time-lost item; i.e., missing half the scheduled work time or more

- *Performance problems*: a score of 3 or more on the SAS performance adequacy item; that is, at least moderate impairment or inadequate productivity at least half the scheduled time

- *Interpersonal problems*: a score of 4 or more on the SAS friction item; i.e., many arguments or significant interpersonal conflicts with co-workers or supervisors; moderate friction or significant avoidance of social contact at work

- *Poor overall functioning*: a mean score of 2 or more on these three functional SAS items

- *Unemployment*

Source: Mintz, J., Mintz, L. I., Arruda, M. J., & Hwang, S. S. (1992). Treatments of depression and the functional capacity to work. *Archives of General Psychiatry, 49,* 761–768. Reprinted with permission from the American Medical Association.

---

upset at work); and interest (lack or loss of interest in the job). As with the functional items, average scores above 2 were considered to reflect affective impairment. These two measures were then used to evaluate the effects of treatments of depression on work impairment.

TREATMENT RESULTS AND WORK OUTCOMES

Major depressive episodes nearly always reduce social, occupational, and interpersonal functioning to some degree, but functioning usually returns to the premorbid level between episodes if the episodes remit completely (Depression Guideline Panel, 1993).

Table 11.6
SAS-BASED CRITERIA FOR
AFFECTIVE WORK IMPAIRMENT

Patients were operationally defined as affectively work impaired if they obtained a mean score of 2 or more on the following three items:

• *Feelings of inadequacy at work*: does not always feel adequate or able to handle things at work; ashamed of work once or twice

• *Feelings of distress at work*: a little distressed at work, or distressed some of the time

•*Lack of interest in work*: only somewhat interested in work or uninterested some of the time

Source: Mintz, J., Mintz, L. I., Arruda, M. J., & Hwang, S. S. (1992). Treatments of depression and the functional capacity to work. *Archives of General Psychiatry, 49,* 761–768. Reprinted with permission from the American Medical Association.

Table 11.7 presents data on SAS-based functional work impairment and depression symptom outcome from six of the treatment research projects analyzed. It is based only on actively treated clients and excludes clients treated with placebo. Work-outcome results are displayed separately for patients who met symptom-remission criteria at treatment termination and for those who did not. Work outcomes were consistently better among clients whose depression remitted. Across the studies, the odds that a client would remain functionally impaired at the end of treatment were nearly 3 times greater if depressive symptoms had not remitted (the pooled-odds ratio was 2.9, p < 0.0001). Note, however, that on average, only approximately 55% of clients achieved symptomatic remission. At least in this type of context, there seems to be an upper limit on the extent to which work restoration could occur.

Table 11.7 also reveals that work outcomes tend to be steadily better as the duration of treatment increases, even if symptoms do not remit completely. Although it seems that this occurs because the likelihood of symptomatic recovery

Table 11.7
POSTTREATMENT WORK IMPAIRMENT, SYMPTOM REMISSION, AND TREATMENT DURATION

Project	Treatment Duration (weeks)	Symptom Remission (%)	Posttreatment Work Impairment Rates In:		
			Remitted Patients (%)	Unremitted Patients (%)	All Patients (%)
Prusoff/Weissman[1]	4	55	57	79	67
Atypical[2]	6	64	36	63	45
Jarrett et al.[3]	10	50	33	50	42
Murphy et al.[4]	12	64	31	67	44
NIMH[5]	16	59	8	18	12
MTRD[6]	39	64	9	–	–

Notes:

1. Prusoff, B. A., & Weissman, M. M. (1981). Pharmacologic treatment of anxiety in depressed outpatients. In D. F. Klein & J. G. Rabkin (Eds.), *Anxiety: New research and changing concepts* (pp. 341-353).
2. Stewart, J. W., Quitkin, F. M., McGrath, P. J., Rabkin, J. G., Markowitz, J. S., Tricamo, E., & Klein, D. F. (1988). Social Functioning in chronic depression: Effect of 6 weeks of antidepressant treatment. *Psychiatry Research, 25,* 213-222.
3. Jarrett, R. B., Rush, A. J., Khatami, M., & Roffwarg, H. P. (1990). Does the pretreatment polysomnogram predict response to cognitive therapy in de pressed outpatients? A preliminary report. *Psychiatry Research, 33,* 285-299.
4. Murphy, G. E., Simons, A. D., Wetzel, R. D., & Lustman, P. J. (1984). Cognitive therapy and pharmacotherapy: Singly and together in the treatment of depression. *Archives of General Psychiatry, 41,* 33-41.
5. Elkin, I., Shea, M. T., Watkins, J. T., Imber, S. D., Sotsky, S. M., Collins, J. F., Glass, D. R., Pilkonis, P. A., Leber, W. R., Docherty, J. P., Ficster, S. J., & Parloff, M. B. (1989). National Institute of Mental Health Treatment of Depression Collaborative Research Program: General effectiveness of treatments. *Archives of General Psychiatry, 46,* 971-982.
6. Frank, E., Kupfer, D. J., Perel, J. M., Cornes, C., Jarrett, D. B., Mallinger, A. G., Thase, M. E., McEachran, A. B., & Grochocinski, V. J. (1990). Three-year outcomes for maintenance therapies in recurrent depression. *Archives of General Psychiatry, 47,* 1093-1099.

• *Logistic regression effects for study duration (c^2=27.11, df=1, p<0.001) and symptom remission status (c^2=10.65, df=1, p<0.002) are statistically significant; placebo-treated patients were excluded.*

Source: Mintz, J., Mintz, L. I., Arruda, M. J., & Hwang, S. S. (1992). Treatments of depression and the functional capacity to work. *Archives of General Psychiatry, 49,* 761-768. Reprinted with permission from the American Medical Association.

increases with an increased duration of treatment, this is not the case. In fact, as shown in Table 11.7, symptom remission rates were quite comparable in "very short" and "very long" treatment studies (e.g., 64% in both a 6-week study of acute treatment [Quitkin et al., 1989; Stewart et al., 1988] and a 9-month maintenance design [Frank et al., 1990; Frank, Kupfer, & Perel, 1989]). These results support the conclusion of Giller and associates (Davidson et al., 1988; Giller et al., 1988) that, based on a longitudinal follow-up design, symptom improvements often occur more rapidly than improvements in the area of work. The lag in work recovery is also consistent with the findings of Weissman, Klerman, Paykel, Prusoff, and Hanson (1974) in an 8-month maintenance study: the effects of treatment on social adjustment may not be evident for at least 6–8 months. The data presented suggest that although the odds of full symptomatic remission are nearly as good in a 4–6-week medication trial as in a 9-month maintenance project, the odds of achieving work recovery steadily improve and may not plateau before 6 months or more.

It is well established and widely known that many effective treatments of depression exist (Depression Guideline Panel, 1993). Because work impairment in depressed clients is intimately tied to symptom severity, it seems obvious that effective symptomatic treatments would also restore work effectiveness. However, this may not be true. For example, relapses and recurrences, as well as the residual symptoms associated with some chronic depressions, might result in demoralization or disrupt the work history such that reentry into the work place would be difficult.

We evaluated this question empirically by analyzing work-outcome data from four controlled studies that contrasted the effects of the tricyclic antidepressants imipramine (Tofranil) and nortriptyline (Aventyl, Pamelor) (Elkin et al., 1989; Murphy et al., 1984; Quitkin et al., 1989; Stewart et al., 1988) or the monoamine oxidase inhibitors phenelzine (Nardil) and isocarboxazid (Marplan) (Davidson et al., 1988; Giller et al., 1988; Quitkin et al., 1989; Stewart et al., 1988) with placebo, and two

Table 11.8

DIRECT COMPARISONS OF MEDICATION, PSYCHOTHERAPY, AND
PLACEBO IN FIVE CONTRIBUTING PROJECTS

| | | | *Posttreatment Work Impairment Rates* | | *Standardized Effect Size (h)†* | |
| | | | | | Drug Versus: | |
Project	N	Drug	Psychotherapy	Placebo	Psychotherapy	Placebo
Atypical[1]	60	45%	—	81%	—	0.77
Giller et al.[2]	39	50%	—	82%	—	0.69
NIMH[3]	51	0%	16%	10%	0.77	0.59
Murphy et al.[4]	16	13%	75%	—	1.36	—
Fawcett et al.[5]	24	0%	—	42%	—	1.39

Notes:

1. Stewart, J. W., Quitkin, F. M., McGrath, P. J., Rabkin, J. G., Markowitz, J. S., Tricamo, E., & Klein, D. F. (1988). Social Functioning in chronic depression: Effect of 6 weeks of antidepressant treatment. *Psychiatry Research, 25,* 213–222.
2. Giller, E. L., Bialos, D., Riddle, M. A., & Waldo, M. C. (1988). MAOI treatment response: Multiaxial assessment. *Journal of Affective Disorders, 14,* 171–175.
3. Elkin, I., Shea, M. T., Watkins, J. T., Imber, S. D., Sotsky, S. M., Collins, J. F., Glass, D. R., Pilkonis, P. A., Leber, W. R., Docherty, J. P., Ficster, S. J., & Parloff, M. B. (1989). National Institute of Mental Health Treatment of Depression Collaborative Research Program: General effectiveness of treatments. *Archives of General Psychiatry, 46,* 971–982.
4. Murphy, G. E., Simons, A. D., Wetzel, R. D., & Lustman P. J. (1984). Cognitive therapy and pharmacotherapy: Singly and together in the treatment of depression. *Archives of General Psychiatry, 41,* 33–41.
5. Fawcett, J., Clark, D. C., Aagesen, C. A., Pisani, V. D., Tilkin, J. M., Sellers, D., McGuire, M., & Gibbons, R. D. (1987). A double-blind, placebo-controlled trial of lithium carbonate therapy for alcoholism. *Archives of General Psychiatry, 44,* 248–256.

• †*Cohen's* h *is a standardized index of effect size; an* h *of 0.50 is "medium" and an* h *of 0.80 is "large." (Cohen, 1988)*
• *Cochran-Mantel-Haenszel (CMH)* c^2 *for medication-placebo contrast, stratifying by study is equivalent to 16.25, df=1, p<0.001; CMH* c^2 *for medication-psychotherapy, stratifying by study is equivalent to 7.11, df=1, p=0.008.*

Source: Mintz, J., Mintz, L. I., Arruda, M. J., & Hwang, S. S. (1992). Treatments of depression and the functional capacity to work. *Archives of General Psychiatry, 49,* 761–768. Reprinted with permission from the American Medical Association.

of which directly compared psychotherapy with medication (Elkin et al., 1989; Murphy et al., 1984). One of these latter studies also contrasted psychotherapy with placebo treatment (Elkin et al., 1989). Some results from these various projects, summarized previously by Mintz, Mintz, Arruda, and Hwang

(1992), appear in Table 11.8. Restoration of work capacity was more rapid with medication than with either placebo or psychotherapy. Of course, the fact that response to drugs may be somewhat faster for many clients is of little value to the client who either cannot, or will not, take drugs. Also, outcomes with psychotherapeutic modalities were somewhat variable. One possibility is that this kind of treatment may be more difficult to deliver consistently from site to site than drug treatment. Psychotherapy and placebo were comparable in the study that addressed this issue. However, the placebo condition in that study was a very active and supportive intervention.

Relapse and Recurrence:

We also analyzed follow-up data from several studies on the effects of relapse and recurrence on work outcomes. Three independent studies using different intervals, follow-up protocols, and measures indicated that recurrence or relapse during follow-up virtually eliminated any short-term benefits associated with remission during acute treatment (Glick et al., 1985; Murphy et al., 1984; Rehm et al., 1987; Spencer et al., 1988). In the study conducted by Rehm and associates (1987), for example, only 5% of clients who remained stable during the entire follow-up period reported significant negative work events at follow-up, compared with 44% of those who either failed to respond initially or relapsed within 6 months ($c^2=9.42$, $p<0.002$). In another study involving the treatment of severely depressed patients in a hospital setting with 1½ years follow-up, 67% of the patients who avoided relapse during follow-up had a good work outcome, versus only 17% of those who relapsed ($\chi^2=4.00$, $p=0.046$) (Glick et al., 1985; Spencer et al., 1988). Results were more impressive in this study using an outcome index that combined symptom remission at treatment termination with relapse during follow-up. A total of 78% of the patients who achieved remission and avoided relapse had good work outcomes, versus only 22% of those who experienced continuing symptoms or required rehospitalization ($\chi^2=5.56$, $p<0.02$).

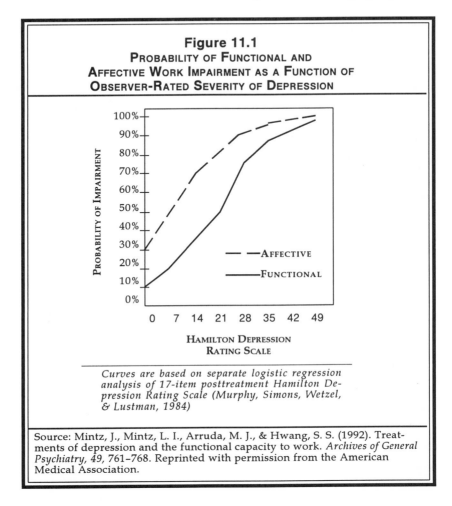

Figure 11.1
PROBABILITY OF FUNCTIONAL AND
AFFECTIVE WORK IMPAIRMENT AS A FUNCTION OF
OBSERVER-RATED SEVERITY OF DEPRESSION

Curves are based on separate logistic regression analysis of 17-item posttreatment Hamilton Depression Rating Scale (Murphy, Simons, Wetzel, & Lustman, 1984)

Source: Mintz, J., Mintz, L. I., Arruda, M. J., & Hwang, S. S. (1992). Treatments of depression and the functional capacity to work. *Archives of General Psychiatry, 49,* 761–768. Reprinted with permission from the American Medical Association.

The Severity of Depression:

Figure 11.1 displays the relations among affective work impairment, functional work impairment, and the severity of depression based on the observer-rated Hamilton Depression Rating Scale. Affective impairment is characteristic of milder levels of depression, whereas functional impairment becomes likely only at moderate-to-severe levels of depression. For example, at Hamilton Depression Rating Scale scores as low as 8 (7 is the conventional cutoff for normal functioning), the model suggests that more than 50% of depressed clients would show affective impairment. In contrast, functional work impairment would not be reached until Hamilton Depression Rating Scale scores were 18 or higher. In clinical terms, the likelihood that a client would experience affective work impairment increased most dramatically as he or she entered the "dysthymic" or "minor" depression range of severity. Comparable increases in functional impairment occurred in the "moderately to severely depressed" range. A Hamilton Depression Rating Scale above 30 indicates that little additional impairment of either type would be expected.

PREVENTIVE INTERVENTIONS

Because of the reciprocal interplay of depression and work impairment, preventive interventions that actually forestall depression, lost work time, and diminished productivity may be cost effective. Employee-assistance programs, which exist in many corporations, might offer ongoing self-screening for depression among the workforce. By using measures that tap job satisfaction, confidence, and enjoyment of work, as well as prodromal symptoms of depression, firms might be able to identify persons who are entering a risk period for a depressive episode. Such persons could then be given information about depression and resources for diagnosis and treatment. Conversely, persons who become involuntarily unemployed (e.g., due to reductions in the work force) and are thus at high risk of developing depression could receive training in job-finding skills and other social support. In fact, a controlled study of this type of preventive intervention reported a significant reduction in depressive morbidity (Caplan et al., 1989).

CONCLUSION

It is essential to be careful when extrapolating from clinical research to practice. Every clinical study has significant limitations that constrain both its scientific validity and its applicability to real-world practice. Clinical samples are highly selective. Research treatment protocols are usually very constrained and thus may not represent the ebb and flow of actual clinical practice. Staffing patterns, assessment instruments and schedules, and all aspects of clinical research procedures probably diverge considerably from everyday practice. Nevertheless, firm scientific evidence (when available) remains the best foundation for general clinical practice, and the scientific method provides the best mechanism for reliable advances in the state of the art.

REFERENCES

Anthony, W. A., & Jansen, M. (1984). Predicting the vocational capacity of the chronically mentally ill. *American Psychology, 39*, 537–544.

Beck, A. T., Ward, C. H., Mendelson, M., Mock, J., & Erbaugh, J. (1961). An inventory for measuring depression. *Archives of General Psychiatry, 4*, 561–571.

Broadhead, W. E., Blazer, D. G., George, L. K., & Tse, C. K. (1990). Depression, disability days, and days lost from work in a prospective epidemiologic survey. *Journal of the American Medical Association, 264*, 2524–2528.

Caplan, R. D., Vinokur, A. D., Price, R. H., & van Ryn, M. (1989). Job seeking, reemployment, and mental health: A randomized field experiment in coping with job loss. *Journal of Applied Psychology, 74*, 759–769.

Clark, D. C., & Fawcett, J. (1989). Does lithium carbonate therapy for alcoholism deter relapse drinking? In M. Galanter (Ed.), *Recent developments in alcoholism* (Vol. 7, pp. 315-328). New York: Plenum Press.

Cohen, J. (1988). *Statistical power analysis for the behavioral sciences.* Hillsdale, NJ: Lawrence Erlbaum Associates.

Cook, J. A., Bond, G. R., Hoffschmidt, S. J., Jonas, E. A., Razzano, L., & Weakland, R. (1992). *Assessing vocational performance among persons with severe mental illness.* Chicago, IL: Thresholds National Research and Training Center.

Davidson, J. R. T., Giller, E. L., Zisook, S., & Overall, J. E. (1988). An efficacy study of isocarboxazid and placebo in depression, and its relationship to depressive nosology. *Archives of General Psychiatry, 45,* 120–127.

Depression Guideline Panel. (1993). *Depression in primary care: Detection and diagnosis.* (Technical report, Vol. 1, Issue 5, pp. 21, 23). Rockville, MD: U.S. Department of Health and Human Services, Public Health Service Agency for Health Care Policy and Research.

Dew, M. A., Bromet, E. J., Schulberg, H. C., Parkinson, D. K., & Curtis, E. C. (1991). Factors affecting service utilization for depression in a white collar population. *Social Psychiatry and Psychiatric Epidemiology, 26,* 230–237.

Elkin, I., Shea, M. T., Watkins, J. T., Imber, S. D., Sotsky, S. M., Collins, J. F., Glass, D. R., Pilkonis, P. A., Leber, W. R., Docherty, J. P., Ficster, S. J., & Parloff, M. B. (1989). National Institute of Mental Health Treatment of Depression Collaborative Research Program: General effectiveness of treatments. *Archives of General Psychiatry, 46,* 971–982.

Fawcett, J., Clark, D. C., Aagesen, C. A., Pisani, V. D., Tilkin, J. M., Sellers, D., McGuire, M., & Gibbons, R. D. (1987). A double-blind, placebo-controlled trial of lithium carbonate therapy for alcoholism. *Archives of General Psychiatry, 44,* 248–256.

Frank, E., Kupfer, D. J., & Perel, J. M. (1989). Early recurrence in unipolar depression. *Archives of General Psychiatry, 46,* 397–400.

Frank, E., Kupfer, D. J., Perel, J. M., Cornes, C., Jarrett, D. B., Mallinger, A. G., Thase, M. E., McEachran, A. B., & Grochocinski, V. J. (1990). Three-year outcomes for maintenance therapies in recurrent depression. *Archives of General Psychiatry, 47,* 1093–1099.

Giller, E. L., Bialos, D., Riddle, M. A., & Waldo, M. C. (1988). MAOI treatment response: Multiaxial assessment. *Journal of Affective Disorders, 14,* 171–175.

Glick, I. D., Clarkin, J. F., Spencer, J. H., Haas, G., Lewis, A. B., Peyser, J., DeMane, N., Good-Ellis, M., Harris, E., & Lestelle, V. (1985). A controlled evaluation of inpatient family intervention, I: Preliminary results of the 6-month follow-up. *Archives of General Psychiatry, 42,* 882–886.

Glynn, et al. (1992). Schizophrenic symptoms, work adjustment, and behavioral family therapy. *Rehabilitative Psychology, 37,* 323–334.

Greenberg, P. E., Stiglin, L. E., Finkelstein, S. N., & Berndt, E. R. (1993). The economic burden of depression in 1990. *Journal of Clinical Psychiatry, 54,* 405–418.

Hagen, D. G. (1983). The relationship between job loss and physical and mental illness. *Hospital and Community Psychiatry, 34,* 438–441.

Hamilton, M. (1960). A rating scale for depression. *Journal of Neurology, Neurosurgery, and Psychiatry, 23,* 56–62.

Jarrett, R. B., Rush, A. J., Khatami, M., & Roffwarg, H. P. (1990). Does the pretreatment polysomnogram predict response to cognitive therapy in depressed outpatients? A preliminary report. *Psychiatry Research, 33,* 285–299.

Liberman, R. P. (1989). *Psychiatric symptoms and the functional capacity for work* (Provisional final report for Research Grant No. 10-P-98193-9004). Baltimore, MD: Social Security Administration.

Massel, et al. (1990). Evaluating the capacity to work of the mentally ill. *Psychiatry, 53,* 31–41.

Mintz, J., Mintz, L. I., Arruda, M. J., & Hwang, S. S. (1992). Treatments of depression and the functional capacity to work. *Archives of General Psychiatry, 49,* 761–768.

Mintz, J., Mintz, L. I., & Phipps, C. (1992). Treatments of mental disorders and the functional capacity to work. In R. P. Liberman (Ed.), *Handbook of psychiatric rehabilitation* (pp. 290-316). New York: Macmillan.

Murphy, G. E., Simons, A. D., Wetzel, R. D., & Lustman P. J. (1984). Cognitive therapy and pharmacotherapy: Singly and together in the treatment of depression. *Archives of General Psychiatry, 41,* 33–41.

Prusoff, B. A., & Weissman, M. M. (1981). Pharmacologic treatment of anxiety in depressed outpatients. In D. F. Klein & J. G. Rabkin (Eds.), *Anxiety: New research and changing concepts* (pp. 341-353). New York: Raven Press.

Quitkin, F. M., McGrath, P. J., Stewart, J. W., Harrison, W., Wager, S., Nunes, E., Rabkin, J. G., Tricamo, E., & Klein, D. F. (1989). Phenelzine and imipramine in mood-reactive depressives: Further delineation of the syndrome of atypical depression. *Archives of General Psychiatry, 46,* 787–793.

Rehm, L. P., Kaslow, N. J., & Rabin, A. S. (1987). Cognitive and behavioral targets in a self-control therapy program for depression. *Journal of Consulting and Clinical Psychology, 55,* 60–67.

Schooler, N., Hogarty, G., & Weissman, M. (1979). Social Adjustment Scale II. In W. A. Hargreaves, C. C. Attkisson, & J. E. Sorenson (Eds.), *Resource materials for community mental health program evaluators* (Publication [ADM] 79328, pp. 290-203). Rockville, MD: U.S. Department of Health, Education, and Welfare.

Spencer, J. H., Jr., Glick, I. D., Haas, G. L., Clarkin, J. F., Lewis, A. B., Peyser, J., DeMane, N., Good-Ellis, M., Harris, E., & Lestelle, V. (1988). A randomized clinical trial of inpatient family intervention, III: Effects at 6-month and 18-month follow-ups. *American Journal of Psychiatry, 145,* 1115–1121.

Stewart, J. W., Quitkin, F. M., McGrath, P. J., Rabkin, J. G., Markowitz, J. S., Tricamo, E., & Klein, D. F. (1988). Social functioning in chronic depression: Effect of six weeks of antidepressant treatment. *Psychiatry Research, 25,* 213–222.

Stewart, A., Greenfield, S., Hays, R., Wells, K., Rogers, W., Berry, S., McGlynn, E., & Ware, J. (1989). Functional status and well-being of patients with chronic conditions: Results from the medical outcomes study. *Journal of the American Medical Association, 262,* 907–913.

Ware, J. E., & Sherbourne, C. D. (1992). The MOS 36-item short-form health survey (SF-36), I: Conceptual framework and item selection. *Medical Care, 30,* 473–483.

Weissman, M. M., & Bothwell, S. (1976). Assessment of social adjustment by patient self-report. *Archives of General Psychiatry, 31,* 37–42.

Weissman, M. M., Bruce, M. L., Leaf, P. H., Florio, L. P., & Holzer, C. (1991). Affective disorders. In L. N. Robins & D. A. Regier (Eds.), *Psychiatric disorders in America: The epidemiologic catchment area study* (pp. 53-80). New York: Free Press.

Weissman, M. M., Klerman, G. L., Paykel, E. S., Prusoff, B. A., & Hanson, B. (1974). Treatment effects on the social adjustment of depressed patients. *Archives of General Psychiatry, 30,* 771-778.

Weissman, M. M., & Paykel, E. S. (1974). *The depressed woman: A study of social relationships.* Chicago, IL: University of Chicago Press.

Weissman, M. M., Prusoff, B. A., Thompson, W. D., Harding, P. S., & Myers, J. K. (1978). Social adjustment by self-report in a community sample and in psychiatric outpatients. *Journal of Nervous and Mental Disease, 166,* 317-326.

Wells, K., Stewart, A., Hays, R., Burnham, A., Rogers, W., Daniels, M., Berry, S., Greenfield, S., & Ware, J. (1989). The functioning and well-being of depressed patients: Results of the medical outcomes study. *Journal of the American Medical Association, 262,* 914-919.

AUTHORS' AFFILIATIONS

Dr. J. Mintz is Professor, Department of Psychiatry and Biobehavioral Sciences, UCLA School of Medicine; Research Psychologist, West Los Angeles Veterans Affairs Medical Center; and Chief, Methodology and Statistical Services Unit, Clinical Research Center for the Study of Schizophrenia, Los Angeles, CA.

Dr. L. Mintz is Assistant Research Psychologist, Department of Psychiatry and Biobehavioral Sciences, UCLA School of Medicine, Los Angeles, CA.

Ms. Robertson [formerly Arruda] is a Research Associate, Department of Psychiatry and Biobehavioral Sciences, UCLA School of Medicine, Los Angeles, CA.

Dr. Liberman is Professor, Department of Psychiatry and Biobehavioral Sciences, UCLA School of Medicine; Director, Clinical Research Unit at Camarillo [CA] State Hospital; Director, Clinical Research Center for the Study of Schizophrenia; and Chief, Treatment Development and Assessment Unit, Community and Rehabilitative Psychiatry Section, Psychiatry Service, West Los Angeles [CA] Veterans Affairs Medical Center.

Dr. Glynn is Assistant Research Psychologist, Department of Psychiatry and Biobehavioral Sciences, UCLA School of Medicine, and Clinical Research Psychologist at the West Los Angeles [CA] Veterans Affairs Medical Center.

12

Psychosocial Therapies for Dysthymia

Robert H. Howland, MD

Dr. Howland is Assistant Professor of Psychiatry, Western Psychiatric Institute and Clinic, University of Pittsburgh School of Medicine, Pittsburgh, PA.

KEY POINTS

- Dsythymia, a mild chronic depressive illness, often develops early in life; the persistence of depressive symptoms can adversely affect both social and vocational development.

- In treating clients with dysthymia, therapists should be flexible, actively engage clients in therapy, develop a strong therapeutic alliance, and show clients how their mood symptoms are linked to their impaired function.

- Interpersonal psychotherapy, social skills training, cognitive therapy, and integrative treatments are all time-limited forms

of psychotherapy that were developed specifically for the treatment of depression and can be useful in the treatment of dysthymia.

- Most important in the treatment of dysthymic clients is to engender hope that the chronic depression they have experienced all their lives does not have to be a way of life; clients can learn that their condition, however chronic, is not immutable and that they now have the option of working toward a meaningful change.

INTRODUCTION

Dysthymia is a chronic depressive illness that afflicts approximately 3% of the general population and as many as 30% of clients attending outpatient clinics. Although dysthymia is considered to be a mild condition (i.e., having fewer symptoms than major depression), significant morbidity and functional impairment can be associated with it (Howland, 1993a). This suggests that the chronicity of symptoms may be as important as their absolute severity. Moreover, dysthymia often develops early in life, and the persistence of depressive symptoms can adversely affect social and vocational development. Dysthymia is thus an important clinical problem that deserves as much attention as any major psychiatric illness.

The concept of dysthymia has generated much controversy among clinicians and psychiatric nosologists (Frances & Cooper, 1981). Because dysthymia is mild, chronic, and often begins early in life, many clinicians regard it as a characterologic trait rather than as a mood state. However, considerable evidence suggests that many of these clients have subsyndromal mood disorders (Howland, 1991, 1993a; Howland & Thase, 1991). An important implication of this formulation is that it broadens the repertoire of treatments that should be considered for such clients. For example, whereas psychotherapy was once considered the treatment of choice, persuasive evidence has now been demonstrated for the effectiveness of antidepressant drugs (Howland, 1991).

Nevertheless, the role of psychotherapy in the treatment of clients with dysthymia should not be minimized. Psychotherapy has been shown to be highly effective for major depression (Robinson et al., 1990). The chronic impairment associated with dysthymia suggests that psychotherapy would be especially useful for this condition. For example, several studies have shown that pharmacotherapy can improve the social and vocational functioning of chronically depressed clients (Koscis et al., 1988; Stewart et al., 1988). However, such improvement is not complete, and residual impairment can be the focus of psychotherapeutic interventions (Markowitz, 1993).

CLINICAL ASPECTS OF DYSTHYMIA

Although dysthymia is related to the mood disorders, there are some important distinctions between dysthymia and major depression that are pertinent to the issue of treatment. The most important characteristic of dysthymia is its chronicity. Often, clients who manifest the illness say they have felt depressed for many years, for much of their lives, or for as long as they can remember. The symptoms of depression wax and wane, but they never disappear for very long, and the risk for major depressive episodes is extremely high. Because the symptoms persist for extended periods, depression literally becomes a way of life. From their perspective, clients see no other way to live: being depressed is normal to them. By contrast, persons suffering from major depression experience an acute change that is distinctly different from their normal state — they feel and recognize they are ill. Clients with dysthymia feel helpless to change their lives and hopeless about the future. Their misery is their destiny (Kraines, 1967).

Another important clinical finding in clients with dysthymia is that many have never been treated previously or have been treated inappropriately with sleeping medication or antianxiety drugs (Ceroni et al., 1984; Keller et al., 1983; Koscis et al., 1986; Scott, 1988a). They often consult their family doctor for problems such as poor sleep, and their depressive condition is not recognized and treated or is nonspecifically treated with sedative-hypnotic drugs. As a result, they experience no relief from treatment and may be pessimistic that any therapy will help. This can then make it difficult — if not impossible — to engage the client in therapy and to develop a hopeful, therapeutic alliance.

Many dysthymic clients have various comorbid conditions,

including other psychiatric disorders, substance abuse, personality disorders, and medical illnesses (Howland, 1993b; Koscis et al., 1990; Markowitz et al., 1992). If these conditions are not recognized or are inadequately treated, their presence can undermine therapy and lead to frustration and failure.

A consistent finding across many studies has been the association of neurotic personality traits with chronic depression (Roy et al., 1985; Scott, 1988a; Scott et al., 1988b; Scott & Eccleston, 1991; Weissman & Klerman, 1977). This psychological construct is defined as a measure of emotional liability or reactivity (Kendrick, 1981). Also, adverse life events are associated with chronicity in depression (Akiskal, 1982; Brown et al., 1988; Scott et al., 1988b; Scott & Eccleston, 1991). These findings highlight the importance of psychological factors and psychosocial stressors in dysthymia. Although psychosocial stressors can precipitate an episode of major depression, their initial role in dysthymia may be to contribute more to the persistence of symptoms rather than to trigger the mood disturbance. Clients with dysthymia may have maladaptive coping skills, perhaps reflecting their degree of neuroticism, such that they react poorly to adverse events. This not only leads to depressive symptoms but also serves to perpetuate the stressors. Thus, an ongoing pattern is set up in which the irresolution of adverse life events leads to the irresolution of depressive symptoms.

Although its clinical symptoms are mild, dysthymia can bring about significant impairment in social and vocational function (Weissman & Akiskal, 1984; Weissman & Klerman, 1977). Clients with dysthymia may be underachievers who do not show progressive success in their work or social lives, or their chronic mild symptoms can lead to a stable level of dysfunction. By contrast, clients with an acute major depression may become temporarily disabled but then recover and return to their previous state of health. This distinction is also evident to family members and significant others. Clients suffering from major depression can be readily recognized as having an illness that requires support and compassion until they recover, whereas clients with dysthymia often engender irritation and impatience in others because the persistence of their condition suggests a personality characteristic rather than an illness (Kraines, 1967).

GENERAL PSYCHOTHERAPY PRINCIPLES IN DYSTHYMIA

Given the clinical issues that are particularly relevant to dysthymia, some general principles are also important in the psychotherapy for dysthymic clients. Special attention must be focused on engaging clients in therapy and developing a therapeutic alliance because of the chronicity of their symptoms and the not-uncommon history of past treatment failures (Kraines, 1967). These clients can be very challenging, and their treatment response is less favorable than for clients with other mood disorders. The therapist must provide reasonable expectations of the therapeutic outcome without giving either false hope or no hope at all. The goals of treatment should be realistic and take into account the client's past history, resources, and personal needs. Psychoeducation about dysthymia can often provide a framework for beginning therapy. It should include information about the various clinical aspects of chronic mood conditions, the impact of the illness on the client's life and that of significant others, and the possible treatment options. By conveying a good understanding of what the client is experiencing and providing a concrete framework for treatment, the therapist will immediately begin to develop an alliance with the client.

A second important principle is the role of the therapist in the process of psychotherapy. Typically, this is determined in part by the theoretical orientation of the therapist. For example, analytical, cognitive, or supportive approaches might dictate particular therapeutic interventions and the degree of activity-passivity by the therapist. However, the client with dysthymia requires more flexibility and patience in the therapist (Kraines, 1967). As noted, the chronicity of the condition often leads to feelings of hopelessness and futility. These clients have little confidence in themselves or others. During the initial stages of therapy, the therapist should be more active, assertive, and directive without dominating or criticizing. The therapist should understand the client's maladaptive behaviors and help him or her to alter them and to learn new skills. More important, the therapist must actively search for areas of success and competence and use these to build momentum in therapy and maintain progress. Later, the therapist can become less active and begin to turn the responsibility back to the client as he or she improves. This principle can be applied with whatever specific therapeutic interventions are used by the therapist.

Finally, therapists working with dysthymic clients should appreciate that their chronic symptoms have become so intertwined with their normal function that depression is a way of life. A major goal of psychotherapy is to show clients how their mood symptoms are linked to their impaired function and that efforts to alleviate their depression can improve their lives (McCullough, 1984). This task is more difficult than it is with a client suffering from major depression, in which the illness and impairment are more easily distinguished from the usual state. With dysthymic clients, psychotherapy should help create a new framework for their lives. By so doing, clients can learn that their condition, however chronic, is not immutable and that they now have the option of working toward a meaningful change. Consideration of alternative ways of life can at least permit the clients to see some possibilities for the future that differ from their hopeless view that what has always been always will be.

INTERPERSONAL PSYCHOTHERAPY FOR DYSTHYMIA

Interpersonal psychotherapy (IPT) is a time-limited form of

psychotherapy that was specifically developed for the treatment of depression (Klerman et al., 1984). IPT primarily focuses on difficulties in the client's interpersonal relationships. This therapy evolved from the finding that depression is often associated with four types of problems: (a) grief, (b) interpersonal role disputes, (c) role transitions, and (d) interpersonal deficits. Interpersonal psychotherapy has been shown to be an effective and easily used intervention in the treatment of major depression (Elkin et al., 1989; Weissman et al., 1981).

Although the use of IPT in treating dysthymia has not been extensively studied, its focus on interpersonal function makes it quite suitable for tackling some problems commonly seen in chronically depressed clients (Mason et al., 1993; Weissman et al., 1981). Adverse life events, losses, and relationship difficulties can sustain depressive symptoms (Akiskal, 1982; Brown et al., 1988; Scott et al., 1988b; Scott & Eccleston, 1991), and these can be directly addressed in IPT. Therapy usually focuses on the "here and now," although past interpersonal problems also are explored and are used to understand maladaptive patterns and to identify areas for change. Interpersonal psychotherapy explicitly defines depression as an illness, which allows the client to assume a "sick" role that requires treatment (Klerman, 1984). Clients are encouraged to examine how their illness has affected their lives and how they can work to become well again. For example, because the dysthymic client's chronic symptoms have become a way of life, changing these symptoms may be viewed as a role transition in IPT (Markowitz, 1993; Mason et al., 1993).

Techniques that are commonly used in IPT include facilitating affect (e.g., expressing repressed anger), encouraging activity and socialization, exploring different options for achieving life goals, examining communication problems, clarifying the client's understanding of his or her interpersonal style, and using the therapy relationship to examine and work through interpersonal problems. The IPT therapist has the flexibility to be directive, offer advice, provide education, and model appropriate interpersonal behaviors depending on the client's needs. However, the ultimate goal is to foster more independent and adaptive functioning by the client so that the therapist can gradually assume a more indirect role as therapy progresses.

SOCIAL SKILLS TRAINING

Social skills training is a short-term, behaviorally oriented form of psychotherapy that was specifically developed for the treatment of depression (Becker et al., 1987). This form of therapy is based on the premise that depression is associated with inadequate interpersonal function. In particular, it suggests that depression results from insufficient positive reinforcement of nondepressed behavior and that important reinforcers for most adults occur in interpersonal activities. Poor interpersonal function can be attributed to many factors, including inadequate or maladaptive social skills, a failure to recognize or accurately interpret social cues, a lack of assertiveness, and a belief that their skills will be ineffective in social situations. Although there appear to be similarities between IPT and social skills training, analyzing and modifying interpersonal behavioral skills are strongly emphasized in the latter. This emphasis may be appropriate for clients with dysthymia whose chronic symptoms may be associated with a lack of interpersonal contacts or with greatly impaired relationships. Some evidence suggesting that social skills training may be as effective as antidepressant medications in chronically depressed clients does exist, although more research is needed in this population (Becker et al., 1987; Hersen et al., 1984).

Social skills training consists of an evaluation of the client's social performance, practical behavioral training of social skills, the use of role playing and practice exercises to reinforce these skills, learning perceptual skills to be used in interpersonal situations, and, finally, teaching clients to monitor their performance and to provide themselves with positive reinforcement. Thus, clients should be able to learn practical skills that will improve their relationships, increase their socialization, and enhance their self-esteem by their interpersonal success.

COGNITIVE THERAPY FOR DYSTHYMIA

Cognitive therapy (CT) is another time-limited form of psychotherapy that was specifically developed for the treatment of depression (Beck et al., 1979). The theoretical basis for this therapy is that depression is invariably associated with automatic negative thoughts about oneself, the world, and the future. This therapy employs various strategies to challenge the validity of such thoughts, thus leading to more accurate and realistic thinking which results in symptomatic improvement of the depression.

Cognitive therapy has been shown to be an effective treatment of major depression (Hollon et al., 1991), and it also has been studied in dysthymia more frequently than other psychotherapies. Uncontrolled studies generally show favorable results in the treatment of chronic depression (McCullough, 1991; Rush et al., 1975; Scott , 1988c; Thase et al., 1994). Some controlled studies have found that the efficacy of CT is comparable to that of antidepressants (Blackburn et al., 1981; Tyrer et al., 1988) and may be superior to supportive therapies (de Jong et al., 1986; Waring et al., 1988). Other studies, however, have not shown CT to be especially beneficial for dysthymic clients (Barker et al., 1987; Fennell & Teasdale, 1982; Harpin et al., 1982). The results from these studies are mixed, although they are encouraging in that even some clients who are refractory to antidepressant medication may respond to CT (de Jong et al., 1986; Rush et al., 1975; Scott, 1988c). Moreover, the use of CT techniques is well suited to address the entrenched and pervasive negative and dysfunctional cognitions in clients with dysthymia.

Cognitive therapy uses specific techniques to focus on the core features of depression (Beck et al., 1979). Cognitive therapists define specific problem areas and teach clients to monitor their daily events to identify situations in which they often feel depressed. Clients also learn to identify the negative and distorted cognitions that automatically arise during such situations and that are linked to the depressed feelings. Then, they examine their beliefs with the help of their therapists, who systematically challenge the beliefs so that clients are able to recognize the distortions and can learn to evaluate thoughts more realistically and accurately. Homework assignments are used to monitor and record the particular problems, situations, automatic thoughts, and feelings that occur outside therapy. Cognitive therapists also encourage clients to pursue various activities that can lead to feelings of pleasure and success and that can counter symptoms such as motivation, isolation, and withdrawal. As therapy progresses, clients should be better able to use their newly learned cognitive and behavioral strategies to accomplish these tasks and to work through different problem areas more autonomously.

INTEGRATIVE TREATMENT OF DYSTHYMIA

In addition to the studies of IPT (Mason et al., 1993; Weissman et al., 1981), social skills training (Becker et al., 1987; Hersen et al., 1984), and CT (Barker et al., 1987; Blackburn et al., 1981; de Jong et al., 1986; Fennell & Teasdale, 1982; Harpin et al., 1982; McCullough, 1991; Rush et al., 1975; Scott, 1988c; Thase et al., 1994; Tyrer et al., 1988; Waring et al., 1988), other psychosocial interventions, such as supportive therapy (Becker et al., 1987; Corney, 1981; Waring et al., 1988; Weissman & Klerman, 1977), dynamic psychotherapy (Bemporad, 1976; Hersen et al., 1984), group therapy (Covi et al., 1974), general psychotherapy (Barrett, 1984), and self-help (Tyrer et al., 1988), have been used with some success to treat chronic depression. However, given the paucity of studies on the treatment of dysthymia, no firm conclusions can be made as to the most appropriate form of psychotherapy. Moreover, studies of the psychotherapy for major depression have not conclusively shown the superiority of any particular therapeutic modality (Robinson et al., 1990). Nevertheless, it is still possible to suggest a psychotherapeutic strategy that can be used in the treatment of dysthymia.

As noted, dysthymia can be distinguished from major depression in several important ways, which can pose a problem for therapists accustomed to dealing with the acute time-limited nature of major depression. As such, it is useful to consider an integrative psychotherapy model that draws on the specific characteristics of different theoretical orientations that can be applied to the unique problems seen in chronically depressed clients. The dysfunction in these clients can be quite pervasive and intractable, affecting all spheres of cognitive, interpersonal, and behavioral function. The most important issue is that such impairment is not merely a change from a normal baseline state; it has assumed an inherent life of its own. Successful therapy uses those techniques from cognitive, interpersonal, social skills, and other psychotherapies that can best and most aggressively confront the myriad problems that contribute to the persistence of the depressive state.

Tailoring Therapy:

In this approach, therapy is tailored to engage and retain clients in treatment; set realistic goals; help clients develop effective problem-solving skills; increase and improve social and vocational activities; and develop increased confidence, mastery, and responsibility in their lives. Of course, the ultimate goal is for clients to assume *a new frame of reference for their lives,* which may entail new roles, new activities, and new relations. It is also important to keep in mind that this change will then mean the loss of their old way of life. Although this change is healthy, clients might feel threatened by the loss of their former stable life and by the uncertainty of the future. Managing this transition is an important task for therapists.

Integrating Other Therapies:

Although psychotherapy can provide important benefits

for clients with dysthymia, it should also be integrated with other therapies to provide a comprehensive treatment program. Antidepressant medications are effective in dysthymia, although less so than in nonchronic depression (Howland, 1991). As discussed, the persistence of depression for prolonged periods (especially early in life) can significantly affect such normal developmental tasks as acquiring social and vocational skills. This suggests that aggressive treatment is needed and that a combined regimen of pharmacotherapy and psychotherapy might be ideal (Markowitz, 1994; Thase & Howland, 1994). Although antidepressants can alleviate many of the depressive symptoms, psychotherapy is needed to rehabilitate the psychosocial deficits (Barker et al., 1987). Some studies of combined treatment in chronic depression demonstrate the advantage of this approach (Barrett, 1984; Blackburn et al., 1981).

Multiple Diagnoses:

Many chronically depressed clients also have associated conditions, such as substance abuse or anxiety disorders, that should not be neglected (Koscis et al., 1990; Markowitz et al., 1992). Substance abuse groups or behavior therapy can be used adjunctively with individual psychotherapy and pharmacotherapy for these clients. In addition, couples, family, and group therapy can be easily integrated into a treatment plan to address other issues. For example, the chronicity of the symptoms in dysthymia can become difficult for significant others to understand and frustrating for them to deal with. Involving significant others in treatment can provide psychoeducation and support for them and can create an environment in which they are able to work with the client rather than undermine the recovery process (Kraines, 1967). Finally, many clients with chronic depression have significant vocational or educational impairment, so a vocational rehabilitation assessment and referral for specialized services may be appropriate.

SUMMARY

In this chapter, I have tried to emphasize some general concepts that are especially important to the understanding of
chronic depression and that can be used to outline a psychotherapeutic approach to its treatment. This is intended to help
clinicians appreciate the distinctions between chronic and
nonchronic forms of depression. Nevertheless, dysthymia is a
heterogeneous condition, and clients will present with different problems and needs. The psychotherapy approach I have
outlined here, using the core techniques from various theoretical models, can address this heterogeneity. In addition, given
the myriad problems associated with chronicity in depression,
integrating psychotherapy with other appropriate therapies
should be seriously considered for all clients. Such an approach can engage and maintain clients in treatment while
providing the best opportunity for a successful outcome. These
clients have struggled with depression for many years, and
this chronic state severely constricts their outlook on life.
Rigid adherence to a limited theoretical or therapeutic orientation may fuel their frustration and hopelessness if it ignores
their specific problems and needs.

REFERENCES

Akiskal, H. S. (1982). Factors associated with incomplete recovery in
primary depressive illness. *Journal of Clinical Psychiatry, 43,* 266–271.

Barker, W. A., et al. (1987). The Newcastle chronic depression study:
Results of a treatment regimen. *International Clinical Psychopharmacology,*
2, 261–272.

Barrett, J. (1984). Naturalistic change over two years in neurotic depressive disorders (RDC categories). *Comprehensive Psychiatry, 25,* 404–418.

Beck, A. T., et al. (1979). *Cognitive therapy of depression.* New York: Guilford Press.

Becker, R. E., et al. (1987). *Social skills training treatment for depression.* New York: Pergamon Press.

Bemporad, J. (1976). Psychotherapy of the depressive character. *Journal of the American Psychoanalytic Association, 4,* 347–372.

Blackburn, I. M., et al. (1981). The efficacy of cognitive therapy in depression: A treatment trial using cognitive therapy and pharmacotherapy, each alone and in combination. *British Journal of Psychiatry, 139,* 181–189.

Brown, G. W., et al. (1988). Life events, difficulties, and recovery from chronic depression. *British Journal of Psychiatry, 152* 487–498.

Ceroni, G. B., et al. (1984). Chronicity in major depression: A naturalistic prospective study. *Journal of Affective Disorders, 7,* 123–132.

Corney, R. H. (1981). Social work effectiveness in the management of depressed women: A clinical trial. *Psychological Medicine, 11,* 417–423.

Covi, L., et al. (1974). Drugs and group psychotherapy in neurotic depression. *American Journal of Psychiatry, 131,* 191–198.

de Jong, R., et al. (1986). Effectiveness of two psychological treatments for inpatients with severe and chronic depressions. *Cognitive Therapy Research, 10,* 645–663.

Elkin, I., et al. (1989). National Institute of Mental Health treatment of depression collaborative research program: General effectiveness of treatments. *Archives of General Psychiatry, 46,* 971–982.

Fennell, M. J. V., & Teasdale, J. D. (1982). Cognitive therapy with chronic, drug-refractory depressed outpatients: A note of caution. *Cognitive Therapy Research, 6,* 455–460.

Frances, A., & Cooper, A. M. (1981). Descriptive and dynamic psychiatry: A perspective on DSM-III. *American Journal of Psychiatry, 138,* 1198–1202.

Harpin, R. E., et al. (1982). Cognitive-behavior therapy for chronically depressed patients: A controlled pilot study. *Journal of Nervous and Mental Disease, 170,* 295–301.

Hersen, M., et al. (1984). Effects of social skills training, amitriptyline, and psychotherapy in unipolar depressed women. *Behavioral Therapy, 15,* 21–40.

Hollon, S. D., et al. (1991). Cognitive therapy and pharmacotherapy for depression. *Journal of Consulting and Clinical Psychology, 59,* 88–99.

Howland, R. H. (1991). Pharmacotherapy of dysthymia: A review. *Journal of Clinical Psychopharmacology, 11,* 83–92.

Howland, R. H. (1993a). Chronic depression. *Hospital and Community Psychiatry, 44,* 633-639.

Howland, R. H. (1993b). Health status, health care utilization, and medical comorbidity in dysthymia. *International Journal of Psychiatry and Medicine, 23,* 211-238.

Howland, R. H., & Thase, M. E. (1991). Biological studies of dysthymia. *Biological Psychiatry, 30,* 283–304.

Keller, M. B., et al. (1983). 'Double depression': Two-year follow-up. *American Journal of Psychiatry, 140,* 689-694.

Kendrick, D. C. (1981). Neuroticism and extraversion as explanatory concepts in clinical psychology. In R. Lynn (Ed.), *Dimensions of personality* (pp. 253-261). New York: Pergamon Press.

Klerman, G. L., et al. (1984). *Interpersonal psychotherapy of depression.* New York: Basic Books.

Koscis, J. H., et al. (1986). Chronic depression: Demographic and clinical characteristics. *Psychopharmacology Bulletin, 22,* 192–195.

Koscis, J. H., et al. (1988). Imipramine and social-vocational adjustment in chronic depression. *American Journal of Psychiatry, 145,* 997–999.

Koscis, J. H., et al. (1990). Comorbidity of dysthymic disorder. In J. D. Maser & C. R. Cloninger (Eds.), *Comorbidity of mood and anxiety disorders* (pp. 317-328). Washington, DC: American Psychiatric Press.

Kraines, S. H. (1967). Therapy of the chronic depressions. *Diseases of the Nervous System, 28,* 577–584.

Markowitz, J. C. (1993). Psychotherapy of the postdysthymic patient. *Journal of Psychotherapy Practice Research, 2,* 157-163.

Markowitz, J. C. (1994). Psychotherapy of dysthymia. *American Journal of Psychiatry, 151,* 1114–1121.

Markowitz, J. C., et al. (1992). Prevalence and comorbidity of dysthymic disorder among psychiatric outpatients. *Journal of Affective Disorders, 24,* 63–71.

Mason, B. J., et al. (1993). Interpersonal psychotherapy for dysthymic disorders. In G. L. Klerman & M. M. Weissman (Eds.), *New applications of interpersonal psychotherapy* (pp. 225-264). Washington, DC: American Psychiatric Press.

McCullough, J. P. (1984). Cognitive-behavioral analysis system of psychotherapy: An interactional treatment approach for dysthymic disorder. *Psychiatry, 47,* 234–250.

McCullough, J. P. (1991). Psychotherapy for dysthymia. *Journal of Nervous and Mental Disease, 179,* 734–740.

Robinson, L. A., et al. (1990). Psychotherapy for the treatment of depression: A comprehensive review of controlled outcome research. *Psychological Bulletin, 108,* 30–49.

Roy, A., et al. (1985). Neuroendocrine and personality variables in dysthymic disorder. *American Journal of Psychiatry, 142,* 94–97.

Rush, A. J., et al. (1975). Cognitive and behavior therapy in chronic depression. *Behavioral Therapy, 6,* 398–404.

Scott, J. (1988a). Chronic depression. *British Journal of Psychiatry, 153,* 287–297.

Scott, J., et al. (1988b). The Newcastle chronic depression study: Patient characteristics and factors associated with chronicity. *British Journal of Psychiatry, 152,* 28–33.

Scott, J. (1988c). Cognitive therapy with depressed inpatients. In W. Dryden & P. Trower (Eds.), *Developments in cognitive psychotherapy* (pp. 177–189). London, England: Sage Publications.

Scott, J., & Eccleston, D. (1991). Prediction, treatment, and prognosis of chronic primary major depression. *International Clinical Psychopharmacology, 6*(Suppl. 1), 41–49.

Stewart, J. W., et al. (1988). Social functioning in chronic depression: Effect of 6 weeks of antidepressant treatment. *Psychiatry Research, 25,* 213–222.

Thase, M. E., et al. (1994). Response to cognitive-behavioral therapy in depression. *Journal of Psychotherapy Practice Research, 3,* 204-214.

Thase, M. E., & Howland, R. H. (1994). Refractory depression: Relevance of psychosocial factors and therapies. *Psychiatric Annals, 24,* 232-240.

Tyrer, P., et al. (1988). The Nottingham study of neurotic disorder: Comparison of drug and psychological treatments. *Lancet, 2,* 235–240.

Waring, E. M., et al. (1988). Dysthymia: A randomized study of cognitive marital therapy and antidepressants. *Canadian Journal of Psychiatry, 33,* 96–99.

Weissman, M. M., et al. (1981). Depressed outpatients: Results one year after treatment with drugs and/or interpersonal psychotherapy. *Archives of General Psychiatry, 38,* 51–55.

Weissman, M. M., & Akiskal, H. S. (1984). The role of psychotherapy in chronic depressions: A proposal. *Comprehensive Psychiatry, 25,* 23–31.

Weissman, M. M., & Klerman, G. L. (1977). The chronic depressive in the community: Unrecognized and poorly treated. *Comprehensive Psychiatry, 18,* 523–532.

13

Alleviating Symptoms of Depression

Mary Ellen Copeland, MS

Ms. Copeland, a counselor, consultant, and educator who specializes in the management of affective disorders, maintains a private practice in Brattleboro, VT.

KEY POINTS

- Counselors should encourage depressed clients to learn about the medical, social, and personal elements of depression.

- Depression may be caused, triggered, or worsened by chronic or acute stress, life issues, or traumatic events. If the client receives counseling while depressed, he or she may prevent recurring depressive episodes.

- It is often useful for clients to use a daily chart to record the subtle changes in mood that usually precede a depressive episode.

- Exposure to full-spectrum light, the use of relaxation techniques,

- daily planning, a proper diet, and exercise alleviate depression.

- Negative thoughts can exacerbate depression. Cognitive therapy and affirmations help clients transform negative thoughts into positive ones.

- Support from family, friends, and health care professionals is essential to the recovery process; it is often helpful for clients to make a list of five people whom they can call on when they need support.

- Effective treatment of depressed clients includes making sure that systems are in place to prevent suicide.

RECOGNIZING SYMPTOMS OF DEPRESSION

When working with clients in the rehabilitation process, the counselor must be aware of symptoms indicative of depression (Table 13.1).

Table 13.1
COMMON SYMPTOMS OF DEPRESSION

• Hopelessness	• Negative attitude	• Irritability
• Uselessness	• Loneliness	• Lack of affect
• Worthlessness	• Isolating behaviors	• Low self-esteem
• Apathy	• Excessive sleep	• Disorganization
• Lack of response	• Insomnia	• Inability to make decisions
• Extreme fatigue	• Poor appetite	
• Lack of motivation	• Excessive eating	• Excessive guilt, embarrassment, or shame
• Physical slowness	• Chronic sadness	
• Low energy level	• Feeling dead inside	• Chronic aches and pains
	• Anxiety	

Copeland, M. (1992). *The depression workbook: A guide to living with depression and manic depression.* Oakland, CA: New Harbinger Publications. Reprinted with permission from New Harbinger Publications, Inc., Oakland, CA.

These symptoms, especially if they continue for more than several days or occur at regular intervals, must be taken seriously. Depression can be a major detriment to the rehabilitation process and, of course, it interferes with basic life enjoyment and attainment of life goals.

MEDICALLY BASED CAUSES OF DEPRESSION

Counseling techniques alone are rarely effective if a biological problem underlying the depressive disorder remains untreated.

A medically based depressive disorder can be caused by chronic or acute disease processes. Depression may be an early symptom of such disorders (Gold & Extein, 1986). The counselor who observes symptoms of depression must refer the client for a complete medical evaluation as soon as possible. Depression caused by illness or some other medical condition is much easier to treat and responds more rapidly to treatment in the earlier stages. Also, because antidepressant medications often take from 3–5 weeks to work effectively (Mondimore, 1990), an early diagnosis would undoubtedly hasten recovery.

Hypothyroidism (thyroid insufficiency caused by diminished production of the thyroid hormone) is a common biological cause of depression that can be uncovered by a complete battery of thyroid tests. Other endocrine or adrenal gland dysfunctions, food allergies, or seasonal affective disorders may also be implicated. It has also been hypothesized that excessive exposure to electromagnetic radiation from electric blankets, water bed heaters, and video screens may be a factor in some depressive disorders (London, 1991).

The depressed client may be unable to make arrangements for a medical evaluation. Therefore, the counselor may have to take a direct approach by contacting health care providers for necessary appointments, arranging transportation, reminding the client of dates and times, and alerting family members and supporters.

A health care *team* is needed for any thorough evaluation. This team usually includes a general practitioner and might include (depending on symptoms, history, and the recommendations of the general practitioner): a psychiatrist, a psychopharmacologist, an endocrinologist, an allergist, and a hospital facility.

Information on health care professionals who are most appropriate for such an evaluation can be found by networking with colleagues and contacting mental health organizations.

Clients rely on members of their personal health care team to:

- Be willing and anxious to know and understand them very well

- Have experience and expertise in treating depression

- Be willing to consider and try alternatives, such as light therapy, exercise, and peer counseling

- Use medication when necessary

- Support, counsel, advise, advocate, understand, and care

MEDICATIONS

It is important for the counselor to understand that clients may fear the side effects of medications. However, medication may be necessary in the short- or long-term to allow the client to begin to control the condition and to enhance the rehabilitation process. Education is the best ally in this process. The client and members of the support team should be well informed about medications before they are administered. Counselors can refer the client and his or her family to resource books, such as *The Physicians' Desk Reference* (Medical Economics, 1996) and *The Essential Guide to Prescription Drugs* (Long, 1996), which are available at most libraries.

Medication and dosage changes must be performed only under the strict supervision of a physician. Moreover, regular tests and physical examinations are absolutely essential for anyone taking psychiatric medications.

Members of the support team must be educated about every aspect of the client's medical treatments so that they can make treatment arrangements and decisions when the depressed client is unable to do so. (Setting up a support team is discussed later in this chapter.)

Hospitalization may be necessary and should be encouraged for any of the following reasons:

- The safety of the depressed client is in jeopardy

- Family members and friends may be unable to provide care

- Drug treatment may need to be monitored initially

- "Time out" in a safe, structured environment would be helpful

- Psychosis or severe agitation is evident

Counselors must be aware of the facilities and programs of the hospitals in their area.

EDUCATION AND EMPOWERMENT

It is important to remind depressed clients that hope does exist. Depression ends; people who experience depression get well and stay well for long periods. In fact, many never have another episode after learning and implementing wellness strategies.

From studying clients who experience depression, it is clear that those who take responsibility for their own recovery ultimately attain the highest levels of stability, wellness, happiness, and control over their lives. Empowering the depressed client to undertake this responsibility, with the assistance of health care and support teams, is a key role of the rehabilitation counselor.

Counselors should encourage depressed clients to learn about the medical, social, and personal elements of depression. This type of education may not be possible when they are in the depths of a depressive episode, but, at other times, the counseling process can emphasize education to alleviate future symptoms as much as possible and to prevent recurrent episodes. Education facilitates appropriate decision making about all aspects of depression, including treatment, lifestyle, education, career, relationships, living space, parenting, and leisure activities. It also enables clients to ask the right questions and to know where to look for answers.

It is often helpful to place depressed clients in touch with educational organizations that publish newsletters for people who experience depression; encourage them to send each organization a postcard requesting a complimentary copy. If the publication is helpful, encourage them to subscribe. They may also decide to attend depression-related workshops and seminars where they can receive input from health care professionals and others who have experienced or are currently experiencing depression.

CHARTING

It is often quite useful to develop and update a daily chart so that the client can respond early and appropriately to the subtle changes in mood that usually precede a depressive episode.

Figure 13.1 is an example of a daily danger signs chart. Because the signs of upcoming episodes vary with each person, page 248 contains an additional chart (Figure 13.2); both may be photocopied and distributed to clients. Work with clients to raise their awareness of their own personal warning signs and use them in the charts.

DIETARY CONSIDERATIONS

What we eat tends to affect how we feel. The following dietary guidelines are helpful for depressed clients to consider (Copeland, 1992; London, 1991):

Figure 13.1
CHART FOR DEPRESSION DAILY WARNING SIGNS

I will be honest with myself in this assessment. If I note that I am showing signs of depression, I will let my support system know, and I will take corrective action that I have learned or that is recommended by others whom I trust.

Date:

SYMPTOMS	Sun	Mon	Tues
Overeating			
Lack of appetite			
Lethargy			
Difficulty exercising			
Fatigue			
Low self-esteem			
Procrastination			
Avoiding crowds			
Irritability			
Impatience			
Insecurity			
Difficulty getting up			
Insomnia			
Poor judgment			
Obsessive thoughts			
Repeating things			
Inability to concentrate			
Destructive risk taking			
Suicidal thoughts			
Paranoia			
Anhedonia (inability to feel pleasure)			

- Avoid eating any one food excessively or exclusively.

- Avoid overeating or undereating.

- Avoid sugar. The clients I studied overwhelmingly reported that sugar exacerbates their depression, makes them hyperactive and foggy, reduces their

---

Figure 13.2

YOUR PERSONAL DANGER SIGNS CHART

I will be honest with myself in this assessment. If I note that I am showing signs of depression, I will let my support system know, and I will take corrective action that I have learned or that is recommended by others whom I trust.

Date:

Symptoms

What to Do Every Day

Medications Taken

---

ability to concentrate, and increases lethargy; some felt "hung over" after consuming sugary foods.

- Limit the amount of caffeine in the diet to a cup of coffee in the morning to get going and a cup of tea in the afternoon; avoid soft drinks with caffeine.

- Be aware of foods that might be affecting clients' moods and use simple avoidance testing for 2 weeks to determine the effects of particular foods on mood.

- Focus on a diet high in complex carbohydrates: rice, potatoes, pasta, whole grain breads, and vegetables; complex carbohydrate foods increase the levels of neurotransmitters (e.g., serotonin) in the brain and thus may function like an antidepressant.

- Avoid high-protein diets and liquid diet drinks.

Counselors should note that clients taking psychiatric medications need to drink plenty of water and avoid fasting.

LIGHT

The importance of receiving full-spectrum light through the eyes is currently a subject of extensive investigation. Exposure to light seems to increase the action of neurotransmitters in the brain, thereby alleviating depression (London, 1991). Counselors should be current with the latest information emerging in this field. Sources of full-spectrum light include sunlight and light from specially manufactured full spectrum bulbs.

Remember these important points about light:

- Advise clients to get outside for as much natural light as possible with glasses off and contact lenses out — even on cloudy days. If a client cannot see well enough to walk without glasses or contacts, he or she should sit outside for 20–30 minutes. However, caution clients to avoid sunlight in the summer months between 10 a.m. and 2 p.m.

- Supplementing light with specially constructed light boxes may be necessary in northern latitudes.

- Distorted spectrum light, such as that found in fluorescent light bulbs, should be avoided; some reports indicate that this form of light makes people uneasy.

- Full-spectrum or Vita-lite has a positive effect on mood stability and overall wellness. (Full-spectrum light bulbs that fit in fluorescent light fixtures can be purchased at hardware and health food stores.)

- Employers should be encouraged to replace fluorescent light bulbs in the workplace with full- spectrum bulbs.

EXERCISE

Exercise helps tremendously in alleviating depression (Copeland, 1992; Dowling, 1991; London, 1991). Better yet, it is arguably the cheapest and most available method for treating depression. Those who experience depression should exercise daily for at least 20 minutes. Any type of exercise they enjoy is acceptable; it need not be strenuous.

RELAXATION

Relaxation techniques have proven very helpful to depressed clients (Copeland, 1992; Davis, Eschelman, & McKay, 1988). Due to the nature and pace of contemporary society, many of us actually need to make a special effort to learn how to relax. However, it is not easy to learn how to relax during a depressive episode. Relaxation usually needs to be learned and practiced when the client is not experiencing full-blown depression, so that he or she will be able to use the methods successfully when depressed or stressed.

Counselors can easily teach relaxation techniques. These strategies can be learned by taking a course, using an instructional video, or practicing the exercises in books, such as *The Depression Workbook: A Guide to Living with Depression and Manic Depression* (Copeland, 1992) and *The Relaxation and Stress Reduction Workbook* (Davis, Eschelman, & McKay, 1988). Structured periods of intense relaxation (10–30 minutes) should be built into the daily schedule.

Counselors should encourage clients to "slow down and take a few deep breaths" or to do a relaxation exercise when they start to feel harried. Relaxation exercises provide a break from depression and can interrupt a downward mood swing.

COGNITIVE THERAPY

Negative and distorted thoughts often instigate a vicious downward spiral. They worsen mood, thereby generating more negative thoughts. Symptoms of depression, such as low self-esteem, low self-confidence, hopelessness, fear, guilt, and embarrassment, benefit from an intensive program of cognitive therapy (changing negative thoughts to positive ones). Jarrett and Rush's chapter on cognitive therapy, included in this volume, provides an excellent overview of the use of cognitive therapy in the treatment of depression. Resources such as *Thoughts and Feelings: The Art of Cognitive Stress Intervention* (McKay, Davis, & Fanning, 1981), *Feeling Good* (Burns, 1980), *The Feeling Good Handbook* (Burns, 1989), and *Cognitive Therapy of Depression* (Beck, 1979) are also valuable guides to this very important work.

Some examples of negative thoughts common in depression — and their positive counterparts — include:

- "I have never accomplished anything" becomes "I have accomplished a great deal." (Working with the client to make a realistic list of accomplishments facilitates this process.)

- "I will never be well again" becomes "I will be well—depression ends. Other people get well and stay well for long periods, and I will, too."

- "No one likes me" becomes "There are many people who like me." (Making a list of friends helps.)

- "I want to die" becomes "I want to live."

Changing negative thoughts to positive ones is often an elaborate, long-term process, but it is well worth undertaking. Remember that cognitive therapy is one aspect of an overall wellness program and should never be considered as a substitute for a complete program of medical and psychological care.

AFFIRMATIONS

Development and regular repetition of affirmations (Table 13.2) may seem like a simplistic concept, but many who experience depression use this technique and find it to be very beneficial. It is noninvasive and free, so it is well worth a try.

In this process, clients make lists of short positive state-

Table 13.2
EXAMPLES OF AFFIRMATIONS

- I enjoy being alive
- I want to live
- I am happy
- I am well

- I am in control of my life
- I am loved
- I trust myself
- I take good care of myself

ments that describe how they would like to feel and how they ideally envision their lives. They develop the habit of filling empty spaces of time (stopped at a street light, washing dishes, upon awakening, bedtime, meditation time) with these affirmations — repeating them again and again. Some people carry lists of affirmations in their pocket or purse, or place them on the refrigerator door. *You Can Heal Your Life* (Hay, 1984) is an excellent reference for affirmations.

CHRONIC OR ACUTE STRESS AND TRAUMA

Depression may be caused, triggered, or worsened by chronic or acute stress, life issues, or traumatic events such as:

- Child abuse or sexual abuse

- Marital problems, especially spousal abuse

- Overwork

- Rejection

- Experiencing or witnessing violence

- War

- Natural or man-made disasters

- Accidents

- Personal loss or tragedy

- Substance abuse (self or family member)

- Stigma

In many of these cases, depression is, in fact, an appropriate emotional response to the circumstance. Intervention at this point may focus on "working through" the mourning period and then putting the events into perspective and resuming a functioning lifestyle.

One of the purposes of counseling at these times is to prevent recurring depressive episodes. The counseling process may be enhanced by:

- Regular peer counseling sessions. The client sets up a peer counseling relationship with someone he or she trusts who is nonjudgmental and willing to listen without giving advice. It helps to have a regular time every week; for example, an hour at 7:00 p.m. on Tuesday. The peer counselors spend equal time sharing and listening to each other.

- Attending a support group for depressed people through which clients can receive encouragement, understanding, and information.

- Using self-help books. In addition to the books listed in the reference section, *I Can't Get Over It: A Handbook for Trauma Survivors* (Matsakis, 1992) is particularly valuable for depressed clients. It validates the trauma of the experience of depression, describes the aftereffects of such an experience, and provides a treatment model that includes numerous self-help exercises.

SUPPORT

Support from family, friends, and health care professionals is essential to the recovery process. However, it is often difficult for depressed clients to gain and maintain a support system because:

- They have low self-esteem

- Their inappropriate behavior embarrasses others

- They are needy and draining

- Their behavior is unpredictable

- They have a hard time reaching out for help

- They become overly dependent on one or a few people

It is often helpful for clients to make a list of five people whom they can call on when they need support. A network of at least five people is essential to prevent wearing any one person out. Also, others are not always available or capable of being supportive. These lists, including telephone numbers, should be posted in convenient places.

Encourage clients to build their support system by:

- Involvement in support groups

- Joining special interest groups

- Attending community events

- Being mutually supportive

- Keeping in touch with friends

- Scheduling contact with peers

- Developing appropriate social skills

Depressed clients need and want love, understanding, acceptance, caring, support, activities, information, protection,

feedback, and monitoring ("reality checks") from these supporters.

PLANNING

Depressed clients often find it very difficult to make plans;
they sometimes cannot even remember the things they enjoy
doing. Accomplishing projects or chores each day, along with
activities they enjoy, helps to enhance motivation.

First, help clients make a list of things they like to do. The
list might include reading a light novel, watching situation
comedies on television, going for a walk, gardening, watching
videos, having lunch with a friend, playing ball, dancing,
painting, shopping, or woodworking. The second list includes
chores they feel should be done, such as washing the dishes,
vacuuming, or making beds. Use these lists, along with the
other components of the wellness program, to help clients
make a plan for the day. Table 13.3 illustrates examples of day
plans that may facilitate functioning in cases of depression.

SUICIDE WARNING SIGNS

Counselors need to be aware of the following suicide warning
signs (London, 1991):

- Talk about committing suicide

- The loss of important person(s) or possession(s)

- Social isolation

- Severe agitation (very dangerous — immediate help
  may be required)

- Alcohol and drug abuse (vastly increase risk for
  suicide)

Table 13.3

SAMPLE DAY PLANS

Day when client is not working

7-8 AM	Get up, shower, eat (cereal with fruit, herb tea)
8-9	Contact support system; arrange people for peer counseling, lunch, and therapy visit; take a walk
9-10	Make beds, vacuum, pay bills
10-11	Peer counseling with close friend
11-12 PM	Work on art project
12-1	Lunch with close friend
1-2	Nap or relax with light novel
2-3	Counseling appointment
3-4	Errands (groceries, renew prescription at pharmacy, library, video store)
4-5	Watch television
5-6	Prepare dinner, eat
6-7	Journal writing
7-9	Watch video with family member
9-10	Read light novel

Day when client is working

7-8	Get up, shower, dress, eat breakfast (bagel with cream cheese, herb tea)
8-8:45	Contact supporters for lunch and evening
8:45-9	Drive to work
9-10	Work
10-10:15	Break, relaxation techniques
10:15-12	Work
12-1	Lunch and walk with member of support team
1-2:30	Work
2:30-2:45	Break, relaxation techniques
2:45-5	Work
5-6	Counseling
6-8	Dinner out with a member of support team
8-10	Watch light video

The beginning of recovery is a very risky time—energy is increased but thought patterns may still be negative.

SUICIDE PREVENTION

To prevent suicide and suicide attempts:

- Insist on treatment of depression early—before it gets out of hand

- Help clients put systems in place, including a suicide support team to prevent suicide (this system should ensure that they are never alone when they are suicidal, even if they insist they want to be alone)

- Educate clients and their family members on the importance of never leaving leftover medication or weapons accessible to clients

- Teach clients relaxation skills, the use of cognitive therapy techniques, and affirmations

- Encourage clients to have pictures of their favorite people in view

- Be sure clients keep appointments with all health care professionals

- Help clients have something planned to which they can look forward

When a client is suicidal, family members, supporters, and health care professionals must take protective action, even if the client refuses such action. It may be necessary to save his or her life.

SUMMARY CHECK LIST

Use the following list as a guide in working with a client with depressive symptoms.

1. Set up a health care team

2. Make sure systems are in place to prevent suicide

3. Make sure that the client:

   a. Has had a complete medical evaluation

   b. Knows the wellness process is his or her own responsibility

   c. Has ongoing education about the illness and has access to additional resources

   d. Identifies early warning signs

   e. Develops and uses planning charts

   f. Considers dietary components

   g. Exercises regularly

   h. Gets full-spectrum light through the eyes

   i. Works on a cognitive therapy program

   j. Develops and uses affirmations

   k. Participates in regular psychological counseling

   l. Has a support team of at least five people

m. Attends a support group

n. Has a regular peer counseling relationship

o. Knows how to make daily plans

REFERENCES

Beck, A. (1979). *Cognitive therapy of depression.* New York: Guilford Press.

Burns, D. (1980). *Feeling good.* New York: William Morrow.

Burns, D. (1989). *The feeling good handbook.* New York: William Morrow.

Copeland, M. (1992). *The depression workbook: A guide to living with depression and manic depression.* Oakland, CA: New Harbinger Publications.

Davis, M., Eschelman, E. R., & McKay, M. (1988). *The relaxation and stress reduction workbook* (2nd ed.). Oakland, CA: New Harbinger Publications.

Dowling, C. (1991). *You mean I don't have to feel this way?* New York: Macmillan.

Gold, M. S., & Extein, I. (1986). *Medical mimics of psychiatric disorders.* Washington, DC: American Psychiatric Press.

Hay, L. L. (1984). *You can heal your life.* Santa Monica, CA: Hay House.

London, W. (1991). *Principles, not principals.* Brattleboro, VT: London Research. (Self published. Available by sending a check for $15 to London Research, 139 Main St., Brattleboro VT 05301.)

Long, J. W. (1996). *The essential guide to prescription drugs.* New York: HarperPerennial.

McKay, M., Davis, M., & Fanning, P. (1981). *Thoughts and feelings: The art of cognitive stress intervention.* Oakland, CA: New Harbinger Publications.

Medical Economics (1996). *The physicians' desk reference.* Montvale, NJ: Author.

Mondimore, F. M. (1990). *Depression: The mood disease.* Baltimore, MD: The Johns Hopkins University Press.

FOR FURTHER READING

American Society of Hospital Pharmacists. (1982). *The consumer drug digest.* New York: Facts on File.

DePaulo, J., & Ablow, K. (1989). *How to cope with depression.* New York: McGraw-Hill.

Matsakis, A. (1992). *I can't get over it: A handbook for trauma survivors.* Oakland, CA: New Harbinger Publications.

Nairne, K., & Smith, G. (1984). *Dealing with depression.* London, England: Women's Press.

Papolos, J., & Papolos, D. (1988). *Overcoming depression.* New York: Harper & Row.

Slagle, P. (1988). *The way up from down.* New York: St. Martin's Press.

14

Decision Making in the Use of Antidepressants: Treatment Considerations

Pedro L. Delgado, MD, and Alan J. Gelenberg, MD

Dr. Delgado is Associate Professor of Psychiatry and Director of Psychopharmacology Research, University of Arizona College of Medicine, Tucson, AZ. Dr. Gelenberg is Professor and Head, Department of Psychiatry, University of Arizona College of Medicine, Tucson, AZ.

KEY POINTS

- The decision to treat a client with an antidepressant medication should follow a careful physical and psychological assessment and diagnosis.

- Medication treatment should be postponed if the diagnosis of major depression is unclear, the symptoms are mild, the risk of harmful consequences of depression is minimal, or the client is strongly adverse to the use of pharmacotherapy.

- Treatment should be viewed as a long-term process involving three stages: an acute treatment phase, a continuation phase, and a maintenance phase.

- Antidepressant drugs have been found to be highly effective in both the acute and maintenance treatment of major depression.

- If a response is obtained in the acute treatment phase, the continuation phase may begin. The primary tasks in this phase include monitoring response, assessing side effects, and establishing compliance; the primary objective is to prevent relapse.

- A recent study investigating the long-term effectiveness of maintenance treatment with imipramine (Tofranil) has become the gold standard for future maintenance studies.

INTRODUCTION

The latter half of the twentieth century has been a period marked by a dramatically increased understanding of the mood disorders. In addition to increasing our understanding of the theoretical basis and pathophysiology of depression, 50 years of clinical research have refined our knowledge of brain function and the mechanism of action of antidepressant medications. Millions of persons who suffer from depression have already received the benefits of this research, with new treatment options being investigated on a daily basis.

With the growth in knowledge and the availability of newer drugs has come an increase in the number of factors that should be considered when selecting appropriate antidepressant medications. This chapter will provide an overview of the decision-making process involved in the selection of appropriate medications for depression and will explore the treatment considerations for each phase of their use.

Initially, it is important to note the limitations in our current concepts of *antidepressant* and *depression*. "Antidepressant" implies selectivity and specificity for depression. However, this is not the case. Antidepressants are effective in the acute treatment of milder mood disorders, such as dysthymia (Hellerstein et al., 1993; Koscis et al., 1987), as well as other mental disorders, such as generalized anxiety disorder (Rickels, Dosning, Schweizer, & Hassman, 1993), panic disorder (Evans, Kenardy, Schneider, & Hoey, 1986; Klein, 1964; Klein & Fink, 1962), social phobia (Versani et al., 1992), obsessive-compulsive disorder (OCD) (Goodman et al., 1989; Pigott et al., 1990), bulimia nervosa and anorexia nervosa (Goldbloom & Olmstead, 1993; Walsh et al., 1984), and posttraumatic stress disorder (Davidson et al., 1993).

Antidepressant drugs affect the core brain systems involved in modulating stress (Chalmers, Lopez, Akil, & Watson, 1993; Henn, Edwards, & Muneyyirci, 1993). The disorders for which antidepressant drugs are effective can be exacerbated by stress (Chrousos & Gold, 1992), suggesting that such medication may simply *restore function*. The high rates of depressive relapse upon discontinuation of antidepressant drugs support this concept (Frank et al., 1990; Kupfer et al., 1992; Prien et al., 1984).

It is increasingly clear that the modern concept of major depression describes a syndrome with many likely etiologic factors. It is highly unlikely that only one type of abnormality, whether inherited or environmentally caused, is responsible for all forms of major depression, dysthymia, cyclothymia, and bipolar disorders. Certain types of cerebral infarcts (Robinson & Chait, 1985), hypothyroidism (Sachar et al., 1985), some of the porphyrias, acquired immunodeficiency syndrome (Perry, 1990), and many types of medications can cause symptoms indistinguishable from those found in depression of unknown etiology.

The limitations of the concept of antidepressants and the heterogeneity of depression argue for the action of these drugs to be compared with the nonspecific anti-inflammatory effects of corticosteroids in the treatment of inflammatory conditions. In this chapter, antidepressants will be defined as those medications for which efficacy has been shown in published clinical studies. *Depression* will refer to the *Diagnostic and Statistical Manual of Mental Disorders* (DSM-IV) definition of major depression (American Psychiatric Association, 1994).

CHOOSING TO PRESCRIBE ANTIDEPRESSANT MEDICATION

The decision to treat a client with antidepressant medication should follow a careful physical and psychological assessment and diagnosis. This can usually be accomplished in one visit, especially if medically relevant, psychiatric, and substance abuse histories are available (American Psychiatric Association Work Group on Major Depressive Disorder, 1993; Depression Guideline Panel, 1993a). Once a diagnosis of major depression has been made, antidepressant medications are usually indicated. In most cases, given the known efficacy and safety of these drugs, treatment should then be initiated with the understanding that the choice of an agent may be significantly affected by presenting symptoms and concurrent psychiatric, medical, or substance abuse diagnoses. Concomitant supportive, educational, or cognitive psychotherapy is usually indicated. When it is appropriate to attempt a trial of psychotherapy prior to medication treatment is an issue beyond the scope of this chapter; however, in general, an indication for psychotherapy is based on clinical presentation, diagnosis, course of illness, past history, and severity.

Several situations call for the initiation of medication treatment as soon as possible. Listed in Table 14.1, they include conditions in which improvement is unlikely without medication treatment, where possible harmful consequences may arise if the depression is untreated (e.g., loss of job or risk of suicide), or where relapse and recurrence are highly likely outcomes. Other situations necessitating medication treatment include a strong family history of mood disorders or major depression with *atypical* features.

Table 14.1
CLINICAL SITUATIONS USUALLY REQUIRING ANTIDEPRESSANT PHARMACOTHERAPY

Major Depression:
- with moderate to severe symptoms
- with potential for suicide or other harmful consequences
- with psychotic features (antipsychotic medication or electroconvulsive
  therapy usually required)
- with melancholia
- when maintenance treatment is planned or relapse likely
- with bipolar disorder (concomitant antimanic drug therapy usually required)
- with prior history of poor inter episode recovery, prior medication response, and failure to respond to psychotherapy
- with obsessive-compulsive or panic disorder

Medication treatment should be postponed if the diagnosis of major depression is unclear, the symptoms are very mild, the risk of harmful consequences of the depression is minimal, or the patient is strongly averse to the use of pharmacotherapy. The most common of these situations occurs when a recent life stress raises the possibility that the presenting symptoms represent a moderate-to-severe form of an adjustment disorder *or* that the depression may be secondary to medical illness, concomitant medication, or substance abuse. The decision to initiate medication treatment in these cases should follow one or two further evaluations.

STAGES OF TREATMENT

Mood disorders appear to be chronic, with high rates of relapse upon discontinuation of drug therapy; therefore, it is important that treatment be conceptualized as a long-term process (Angst et al., 1973; Frank et al., 1990, 1991; Keller et al., 1982; Kraepelin, 1921; Kupfer, 1991; Montgomery & Montgomery, 1992; Prien & Kupfer, 1986). Even though medications restore function, the disease is not cured.

Three stages of treatment have been proposed: an acute treatment phase, a continuation phase, and a maintenance phase (Kupfer, 1991). The stages are defined in relation to the status of symptoms and involve the concepts of treatment response, relapse, remission, recurrence, and recovery (Kupfer, 1991; Prien et al., 1984).

Response refers to a decrease in symptoms following initiation of drug treatment. *Relapse* involves the return of some symptoms of a disease during or upon cessation of treatment. *Remission* refers to a clinically meaningful diminution of the symptoms of a disease. *Recurrence* describes the return of symptoms after a remission. *Recovery* describes a more complete remission, implying the absence or near absence of symptoms.

Acute Treatment Phase:

The acute treatment phase begins with a clinical interview, diagnostic assessment, physical and neurological examinations, and clinical and laboratory studies as appropriate (American Psychiatric Association Work Group on Major Depressive Disorder, 1993; Depression Guideline Panel, 1993a, 1993b). A decision to initiate treatment is based on the presence of diagnostic criteria for major depression or a manic episode. The goals of this phase include: establishing a diagnosis, defining short-term and long-term multidisciplinary treatment plans, selecting the most appropriate medication, titrating the dose to a therapeutic range, monitoring side effects, maintaining compliance, and determining the magnitude and quality of response. During this phase, which lasts 6–12 weeks, clients usually are seen for medication management every 1–2 weeks. If a satisfactory treatment response is achieved, the continuation phase will follow. If a new treatment is initiated, a second acute treatment phase may ensue. An algorithm for decision making has been suggested for antidepressant treatment phases (American Psychiatric Association Work Group on Major Depressive Disorder, 1993; Depression Guideline Panel, 1993b). A modified version is presented in Figure 14.1.

All current antidepressant medications require continuous dosing for an average of 10–21 days before major clinical improvement is evident. This time lag in action is unrelated to the time required to achieve therapeutic doses and is thought to be due to a time-dependent process of neuronal adaptation. For most drugs, raising the dose beyond the usual therapeutic range does not speed up response but rather exacerbates side effects. For some drugs, such as nortriptyline (Aventyl, Pamelor), with so-called therapeutic windows, higher-than-usual doses actually can be associated with a lower rate of response. These facts strongly argue for titration to the usual therapeutic dose range and for monitoring of the response during the first 21 days of treatment.

The rate of dose titration is closely related to a medication's side-effect profile. The most anticholinergic and antiadrenergic

Figure 14.1
AN ALGORITHM FOR THE TREATMENT OF DEPRESSION

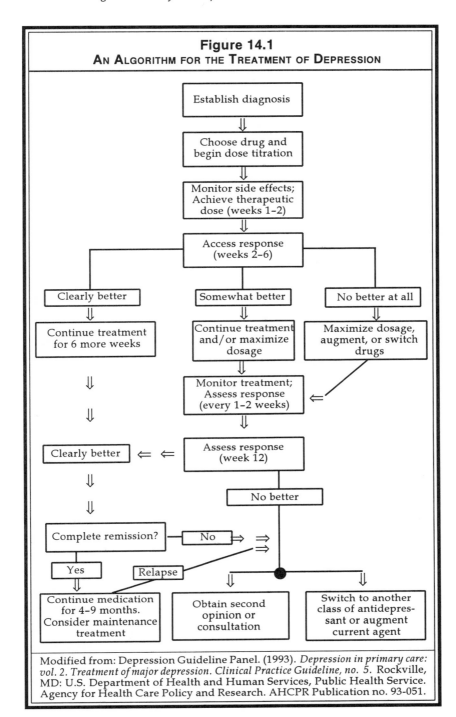

Modified from: Depression Guideline Panel. (1993). *Depression in primary care: vol. 2. Treatment of major depression. Clinical Practice Guideline, no. 5.* Rockville, MD: U.S. Department of Health and Human Services, Public Health Service. Agency for Health Care Policy and Research. AHCPR Publication no. 93-051.

drugs require the most careful titration. It is not uncommon for the clinician to be unable to achieve therapeutic doses of these medications because of the severity of side effects. This is especially true for clomipramine (Anafranil), amitriptyline (Elavil), doxepin (Sinequan), amoxapine (Asendin), and trazodone (Desyrel). On the other hand, for all selective serotonin reuptake inhibitors (SSRIs) except fluvoxamine (Luvox), the therapeutic dose may usually be started at once. Because of nausea and asthenia, most investigators have titrated the dose of fluvoxamine over a 7–14-day period.

Because of the minor side-effect profile associated with SSRIs and the relative lack of routine clinical use of these agents, these medications are frequently used at doses much higher than required. Such administration was common with fluoxetine (Prozac) in the first few years after its introduction; gradually, it became apparent that 20 mg/day was an adequate dose for most clients. Doses of paroxetine (Paxil) and sertraline (Zoloft) are often raised too rapidly. For these drugs, most investigators agree, doses of 20 mg/day of paroxetine and 50–100 mg/day of sertraline are therapeutic. In older clients or in clients who are sensitive to side effects, starting doses of 5–10 mg of fluoxetine, 10 mg of paroxetine, or 25 mg of sertraline are recommended.

Assessment of treatment response should include an evaluation of current depressive symptoms as well as a determination of current level of function. Treatment response is clearly a continuous variable, with some clients having limited symptom relief. Other clients experience a complete restoration of normal function; and others develop a degree of improvement that is better than their prior best level of functioning.

Conceptual guidelines for defining treatment response have recently been published (Prien et al., 1984). The distinction between partial remission and full remission can be important. *Partial remission* involves a treatment response such that the client no longer meets the full criteria for major depression or manic episode but continues to have more than minimal symptoms. *Full remission* is declared when a client no longer meets criteria for major depression or manic episode and has no more than minimal symptoms (Prien et al., 1984). Factors important in assessing therapeutic response are listed in Table 14.2.

Table 14.2
ASSESSING THERAPEUTIC RESPONSE

No longer meets criteria for major depressive or manic episode
Presence or absence of specific symptoms
Level of functioning
Side effects

If, after 3 or 4 weeks, the client has shown no evidence of response, the dose should be titrated toward the maximum recommended dose as tolerated. For tricyclic antidepressants and monoamine oxidase inhibitors, the dose can be increased in 3- or 4-day intervals, but for SSRIs it should be raised in 7–14-day intervals, because most clients respond to the lower dose ranges. If, after a 4–6-week period, the client still has not achieved a partial response, a careful reevaluation of current treatment should be pursued. This involves reassessing the accuracy of the diagnosis, investigating dynamic psychosocial factors, discussing compliance issues with the client, assessing the current dose, and giving consideration to switching the medication treatment or augmenting the current regimen.

If a partial response has been achieved after a 4–6-week period, waiting a full 12 weeks usually results in continued improvement and a full response. If the rate of improvement has reached a plateau after 12 weeks, consideration should be given to changing or augmenting medications. If improvement is continuing, the acute period should be extended until the response has reached a plateau.

Plasma drug levels are most important when assessing the

reasons for a lack of response, when a higher than expected degree of side effects is being encountered, or when toxicity is suspected. Evidence supports the presence of minimum therapeutic plasma levels for desipramine (Norpramin, Pertofrane), imipramine (Tofranil), amitriptyline, and nortriptyline. Nortriptyline appears to have a therapeutic window, with plasma levels above 150 ng/mL being less effective than those between 50 and 150 ng/mL. Plasma levels of desipramine, imipramine, and amitriptyline above 300 ng/mL are associated with a higher risk of potentially dangerous side effects, such as cardiac conduction abnormalities or seizures.

Continuation Phase:

If a response is obtained, the continuation phase begins; it consists of monitoring for completeness of response and side effects. Discontinuation of medication during or before this phase has been completed is associated with a high rate of relapse (Kupfer, 1991; Prien & Kupfer, 1986). Continuation treatment lasts 4–9 months and can be viewed as a consolidation phase. A recent World Health Organization (WHO) consensus meeting suggested 6 months as the minimum period for continuation treatment (Altamura & Percudani, 1993; Kupfer et al., 1992; WHO Mental Health Collaborating Centers, 1989).

The primary tasks of the continuation phase are to monitor response, assess side effects, and establish compliance; the primary objective is to prevent relapse. If maintenance treatment is not planned, medication should be gradually tapered over a 4–6-week period at the end of this phase.

Several factors are associated with a higher risk of relapse and need to be considered before discontinuation of medication is started. Clients with residual symptoms, significant psychosocial problems, or a history of prior relapse or recurrence are at increased risk for recurrence after continuation therapy. Given the high rates of recurrence of major depression, most clients should be strongly encouraged to consider maintenance treatment.

Maintenance Phase:

The majority of clients with a mood disorder will have more than one episode. Recurrence rates for depression are estimated to be at least 50% for clients with one episode of major depression and 80%–90% if the client has had two episodes (Angst, 1990; Kupfer, 1991). Of the clients who have been successfully treated for major depression, 70%–90% will experience a recurrence of illness when active medication is replaced by placebo during a 3-year maintenance phase, as opposed to only 15%–20% of those taking a full dose of imipramine (Prien et al., 1984). In a prospective 10-year epidemiologic follow-up study of young depressed clients, 78% relapsed during the follow-up period (Angst, 1990). These high rates of recurrence and relapse have highlighted the need for consideration of the efficacy of antidepressant treatments in the continuation and maintenance phases of treatment.

Maintenance treatment is thought to be prophylactic, geared toward the prevention of recurrence; however, it is increasingly clear that maintenance treatment is essential for maintaining the response, because the illness — whatever its true nature — persists. Clients with two or more prior episodes of major depression, those with more severe episodes, and those with a risk of suicide should be strongly encouraged to consider maintenance treatment. Clients with multiple mild episodes spaced at long intervals and with complete inter-interval recovery obviously may choose not to use maintenance treatment.

Studies of maintenance treatment have taken on considerable importance in light of recent findings of high rates of relapse and recurrence in clients with relatively uncomplicated major depression following continuation treatment (Frank et al., 1990; Kupfer et al., 1992; Prien et al., 1984). The most studied medication in the maintenance treatment of major depression is imipramine. The recent study by the Pittsburgh group (Kupfer et al., 1992) that investigated the long-term effectiveness of maintenance treatment with imipramine has become the gold standard for future maintenance studies. This study and the earlier studies by the same group (Frank et al., 1990), as well as the study by Prien and colleagues (1984), have made imipramine the drug against which other drugs should be compared. The rate of relapse or recurrence during imipramine treatment is between 20% and 30%, whereas the rate of relapse with placebo approaches 80% over a 1–3-year treatment period. A dosage of imipramine below the usual therapeutic range (150–300 mg/day, plasma level > 150 ng/mL) leads to a higher rate of relapse, suggesting that maintenance treatment should employ full antidepressant doses (Kupfer et al., 1992).

For managing medications, clients should be seen every 4–12 weeks for the first year of maintenance treatment and at intervals of 6–12 months thereafter. The frequency of visits during this phase should be individualized on the basis of psychosocial factors, compliance, and presence of symptoms and side effects. Rates of depressive relapse appear to be higher when antidepressant drugs are discontinued rapidly, compared with a slow 3–4-week taper (Kupfer, 1991; Robinson et al., 1991). Therefore, if medication is discontinued, it should be tapered over a 4-week period.

CONCLUSION

In summary, antidepressant medications are highly effective in the acute and maintenance treatment of major depression. Although the disorders are usually chronic and the vulnerability to the illness remains, most clients can live relatively normal lives with minimal treatment-related side effects.

REFERENCES

Altamura, A. C., & Percudani, M. (1993). The use of antidepressants for long-term treatment of recurrent depression: Rationale, current methodologies, and future directions. *Journal of Clinical Psychiatry, 54*(Suppl. 8), 29–37.

American Psychiatric Association. (1994). *Diagnostic and statistical manual of mental disorders* (4th ed). Washington, DC: Author.

American Psychiatric Association Work Group on Major Depressive Disorder. (1993). American Psychiatric Association practice guidelines: Practice guidelines for major depressive disorder in adults. *American Journal of Psychiatry, 150*, 1–26.

Angst, J. (1990). National history and epidemiology of depression: Results of community studies. In J. Cobb & N. Goeting (Eds.), *Prediction and treatment of recurrent depression* (pp. 1-9). Southampton, UK: Duphar Medical Relations.

Angst, J., et al. (1973). The course of monopolar depression and bipolar psychoses. *Psychiatria, Neurologia, Neurochirugia, 76*, 489–500.

Chalmers, D. T., Lopez, J. F., Akil, H., & Watson, S. J. (1993). Molecular aspects of the stress axis and serotonergic function in depression. *Clinical Neuroscience, 1*(3), 122–128.

Chrousos, G. P., & Gold, P. W. (1992). The concepts of stress and stress system disorders: Overview of physical and behavioral homeostasis. *Journal of the American Medical Association, 267*, 1244–1252.

Davidson, J. R. T., et al. (1993). Predicting response to amitriptyline in posttraumatic stress disorder. *American Journal of Psychiatry, 150*, 1024–1029.

Depression Guideline Panel. (1993a). *Depression in primary care: vol. 1. Detection and diagnosis. Clinical Practice Guideline, no. 5.* Rockville, MD: U.S. Department of Health and Human Services, Public Health Service. Agency for Health Care Policy and Research. AHCPR Publication no. 93-051.

Depression Guideline Panel. (1993b). *Depression in primary care: vol. 2. Treatment of major depression. Clinical Practice Guideline, no. 5.* Rockville, MD: U.S. Department of Health and Human Services, Public Health Service. Agency for Health Care Policy and Research. AHCPR Publication no. 93-051.

Evans, L., Kenardy, J., Schneider, P., & Hoey, H. (1986). Effect of a selective serotonin-uptake inhibitor in agoraphobia with panic attacks: A double-blind comparison of zimelidine, imipramine, and placebo. *Acta Psychiatrica Scandinavica, 73,* 49–53.

Frank, E., et al. (1990). Three-year outcomes for maintenance therapies in recurrent depression. *Archives of General Psychiatry, 47,* 1093–1099.

Frank, E., et al. (1991). Conceptualization and rationale for consensus definitions of terms in major depressive disorder: Response, remission, recovery, relapse, and recurrence. *Archives of General Psychiatry, 48,* 851–855.

Goldbloom, D. S., & Olmstead, M. P. (1993). Pharmacotherapy of bulimia nervosa with fluoxetine: Assessment of clinically significant attitudinal change. *American Journal of Psychiatry, 150,* 770–774.

Goodman, W. K., Price, L. H., Rasmussen, S. A., Delgado, P. L., Heninger, G. R., & Charney, D. S. (1989). Efficacy of fluvoxamine in obsessive-compulsive disorder: A double-blind comparison with placebo. *Archives of General Psychiatry, 46,* 36–44

Hellerstein, D. J., et al. (1993). A randomized double-blind study of fluoxetine versus placebo in the treatment of dysthymia. *American Journal of Psychiatry, 150,* 1169–1175.

Henn, F. A., Edwards, E., & Muneyyirci, J. (1993). Animal models of depression. *Clinical Neuroscience, 1*(3), 152–156.

Keller, M. B., et al. (1982). Recovery in major depressive disorder: Analysis with the life table and regression models. *Archives of General Psychiatry, 39,* 905–910.

Klein, D. F. (1964). Delineation of two drug-responsive anxiety syndromes. *Psychopharmacologia, 5,* 397–408.

Klein, D. F., & Fink, M. (1962). Psychiatric reaction patterns of imipramine. *American Journal of Psychiatry, 119*, 432–438.

Koscis, J. H., Frances, A. J., Voss, C. B., Mann, J. J., Mason, B. J., & Sweeney, J. (1987). Imipramine for treatment of chronic depression. *Archives of General Psychiatry, 45*, 253–257.

Kraepelin, E. (1921). *Manic depression illness*. Edinburgh, Scotland: E & S Livingstone.

Kupfer, D. J. (1991). Long-term treatment of depression. *Journal of Clinical Psychiatry, 52*(Suppl. 5), 28–34.

Kupfer, D. J., et al. (1992). Five-year outcome for maintenance therapies in recurrent depression. *Archives of General Psychiatry, 49*, 769–773.

Montgomery, S. A., & Montgomery, D. B. (1992). Prophylactic treatment in recurrent unipolar depression. In S. A. Montgomery & F. Roullon (Eds.), *Long-term treatment of depression* (pp. 53–72). New York: John Wiley & Sons.

Perry, S. W. (1990). Organic mental disorders caused by HIV: Update on early diagnosis and treatment. *American Journal of Psychiatry, 147*, 696–710.

Pigott, T. A., et al. (1990). Controlled comparisons of clomipramine and fluoxetine in the treatment of obsessive-compulsive disorder. *Archives of General Psychiatry, 47*, 926–932.

Prien, R. F., et al. (1984). Drug therapy in the prevention of recurrences in unipolar and bipolar affective disorders: Report of the NIMH Collaborative Study Group comparing lithium carbonate, imipramine, and a lithium carbonate-imipramine combination. *Archives of General Psychiatry, 41*, 1096–1104.

Prien, R. F., & Kupfer, D. J. (1986). Continuation therapy for major depressive episodes: How long should it be maintained? *American Journal of Psychiatry, 143*, 18–23.

Rickels, K., Dosning, R., Schweizer, E., & Hassman, H. (1993). Antidepressants for the treatment of generalized anxiety disorder: A placebo-controlled comparison of imipramine, trazodone, and diazepam. *Archives of General Psychiatry, 50*, 884–895.

Robinson, R. G., et al. (1991). Continuation and maintenance treatment of major depression with the monoamine oxidase inhibitor phenelzine: A double-blind placebo-controlled discontinuation study. *Psychopharmacology Bulletin, 27,* 31–39.

Robinson, R. G., & Chait, R. M. (1985). Emotional correlates of structural brain injury with particular emphasis on post-stroke mood disorders. *CRC Critical Reviews in Clinical Neurobiology, 1*(4), 285–318.

Sachar, E. J., et al. (1985). Three tests of cortisol secretion in adult endogenous depression. *Acta Psychiatrica Scandinavica, 71,* 1–8.

Versani, M., et al. (1992). Pharmacotherapy of social phobia: A controlled study with moclobemide and phenelzine. *British Journal of Psychiatry, 161,* 353–360.

Walsh, J. I., et al. (1984). Treatment of bulimia with phenelzine: A double-blind placebo-controlled study. *Archives of General Psychiatry, 4,* 1105–1109.

WHO Mental Health Collaborating Centers. (1989). Pharmacotherapy of depressive disorders: A consensus statement. *Journal of Affective Disorders, 17,* 197–198.

Name Index

A

Aagesen, C. A., 219
Ablow, K., 263
Abou-Saleh, M. T., 107, 109
Adams, R. D., 34, 46
Ader, R., 32
Adey, M., 172
Adolph, M. R., 82, 90
Agrell, B., 158, 171
Akil, H., 266, 277
Akiskal, H., 13
Akiskal, H. S., 228, 231, 237, 241
Aldwin, C. M., 148, 171
Altamura, A. C., 274, 277
Andersen, Arnold E., 52, 60, 63
Andersen, G., 42, 46
Andrezejewski, P., 43, 47
Angst, J., 269, 275, 277
Anthony, W. A., 202, 203, 218
Antico, L., 174
Aries, E., 78, 90
Arieti, S., 186, 190, 196
Arruda, M. J., 200, 214, 220

B

Baike, E., 164, 173
Baldessarini, R. J., 35, 46
Barefoot, J. C., 89, 90
Barker, W. A., 233, 234, 236, 237
Barrett, J., 234, 236, 237
Baser, D., 35, 46
Beck, A. T., 128, 129, 132, 133, 134, 139,
    140, 141, 142, 143, 144, 146,
    157, 166, 171, 184, 196, 204,
    218, 233, 238, 253, 262
Becker, R. E., 232, 234, 238
Beckham, E. E., 141, 143
Beckham, J. C., 89, 90
Belsky, J. K., 70, 90
Bemporad, J., 182, 185, 186, 187, 192,
    196, 234, 238
Benowitz, L. I., 35, 46
Berman, J. S., 119, 126
Berndt, E. R., 201, 220
Berne, E., 181, 196

Berry, S., 221, 222
Besedovsky, H., 16, 30
Bialos, D., 209, 219
Bialow, M. R., 157, 176
Bibring, E., 196
Biglan, A., 171
Birtchnell, John A., 180, 181, 183, 184,
    185, 195, 196, 197
Bishop, S., 141, 143
Black, H. R., 98, 109
Blackburn, I. M., 140, 141, 143, 233, 234,
    236, 238
Blalock, J., 17, 32
Blazer, D. G., 148, 149, 150, 155, 171, 175,
    201, 218
Bleuler, E. P., 34, 46
Bolduc, P., 38, 49
Bolla-Wilson, K., 41, 46
Bond, G. R., 219
Boston, J., 41, 46
Bothwell, S., 206, 221
Bourgeois, M. S., 153, 172
Bowen, M., 190, 197
Bowlby, J., 4, 5, 13
Brand, E., 169, 170, 172
Breckenridge, J. N., 157, 168, 172, 177
Breckenridge, J. S., 140, 146
Brink, T. L., 172
Broadhead, W. E., 201, 218
Brody, E. M., 66, 91
Bromet, E. J., 201, 219
Brosse, R., 148, 171
Brown, D. C., 160, 174
Brown, G. W., 228, 231, 238
Bruce, M. L., 69, 91, 201, 202
Bullock, R. C., 183, 197
Burlew, L. D., 87, 91
Burnham, A., 222
Burns, D., 253, 262
Butler, R., 83, 91

C

Cantwell, D. P., 52, 63

Caplan, R. D., 202, 217, 218
Capparella, O., 174
Carboni, P. U., 174
Carman, J. S., 108, 110
Carman, M. B., 84, 91
Ceroni, G. B., 227, 238
Chait, R. M., 267, 280
Chalmers, D. T., 266, 277
Chancellor-Freeland, Cheryl, 27, 31
Charney, D. S., 278
Charpentier, B., 28, 30
Chevron, E. S., 114, 125
Chodoff, P., 184, 197
Chrousos, G. P., 266, 277
Clark, D. C., 209, 218, 219
Clark, E. O., 154, 175
Clarkin, J. F., 220, 221
Clemmons, R., 157, 176
Clingempeel, W. G., 169, 170, 172
Cohen, D., 172
Cohen, H. J., 148, 150, 175
Cohen, J., 218
Cohen, N., 32
Cohen, S., 27, 31
Collin, S. J., 35, 36, 44, 46
Collins, J. F., 219
Conn, D. K., 44, 48
Cook, J. A., 203, 204, 219
Cooper, A., M., 226, 238
Coopersmith, S., 13
Copeland, Mary Ellen, 248, 252, 253, 262
Coppen, A., 107, 109
Corey, M., 85, 88, 91
Cornes, C., 219
Corney, R. H., 234, 238
Costello, C. G., 164, 172
Covi, L., 143, 234, 238
Coyne, J. C., 44, 49
Crary, B., 23, 30
Cupps, T., 22, 30
Curtis, E. C., 201, 219
Czirr, R., 141, 146

D

Dackis, C. A., 96, 101, 109
Daniels, M., 222
Dantzer, R., 16, 30
Davidson, J. R. T., 209, 213, 219, 266, 277
Davis, M., 252, 253, 262
de Jong, R., 233, 234, 238
Dehlin, O., 158, 171
Delgado, Pedro L., 278
D'Elia, L. F., 154, 175
DeMane, N., 220, 221

Dennis, M., 35, 41, 47
DePaulo, J., 263
Derby, J.F., 86, 91
Dessonville, C., 172
Dew, M. A., 201, 219
Dobson, K. S., 140, 144
Docherty, J. P., 219
Dosning, R., 266, 279
Dow, M. G., 171
Dowling, C., 252, 262
Down, M., 140, 144
Downhill,, J. E., 41, 46
Draper, E., 185, 186, 197
Dublin, J. E., 188, 197
Dusay, J. M., 193, 197

E

Ebrahim, S., 35, 46
Eccleston, D., 228, 231, 241
Edwards, A., 29, 31
Edwards, E., 266, 278
Eisdorfer, C., 148, 172
Elkin, I., 140, 141, 144, 209, 213, 214, 219, 231, 238
Emerson, P., 87, 91
Endicott, J., 155, 172
Engel, G., 3, 4, 13
Epstein, S., 13
Erbaugh, J., 157, 171, 204, 218
Eschelman, E. R., 252, 253, 262
Estroff, T.W., 96, 106, 109
Eunson, K. M., 141, 143
Evans, L., 266, 278
Extein, I., 96, 101, 102, 103, 104, 106, 109, 111, 245, 262

F

Faith, R., 24, 32
Falkowski, J., 184, 197
Fanning, P., 253, 262
Farberow, N., 120, 126
Fast, I., 185, 197
Fauci, A., 22, 30
Fawcett, J., 209, 218, 219
Fedoroff, J. P., 48
Feibel, J. H., 35, 41, 44, 46
Felton, D. L., 32
Fenichel, O., 182, 197
Fennell, M. J. V., 233, 234, 238
Ferster, C. B., 163, 164, 172
Ficster, S. J., 219
Fink, M., 266, 279

Holtzworth-Munroe, A., 141, 144
Holzer, C., 201, 222
Holzer, C. E., 157, 176
Hopps, H., 163, 174
Horowitz, M., 168, 174
House, A., 35, 41, 47
Howland, Robert H., 226, 228, 236, 239, 241
Hudson, J. I., 53, 64
Hughes, D. C., 148, 171
Hussian, R. A., 160, 168, 174
Hwang, S. S., 200, 214, 220

I

Imber, S. D., 219
Incalzi, R. A., 150, 174
Irwin,M., 29, 31

J

Jacobson, N. S., 141, 144
Jansen, M., 202, 203, 218
Jarrett, D. B., 219
Jarrett, R. B., 171, 175, 209, 220
Jarrett, Robin B., 140, 142, 144
Jarvik, L. A., 150, 154, 174, 175
Jefferson, J. W., 100, 106, 107, 111
Jensen, L., 88, 91
Johnson-Sabine, E. C., 53, 64
Jonas, E. A., 219
Jones, J., 87, 91
Jones, L., 35, 47

K

Kaltreider, N., 168, 174
Kaslow, N. J., 209, 221
Katz, I. R., 150, 176
Keller, M. B., 94, 112, 227, 239, 269, 278
Kelly, K. W., 16, 30
Kenardy, J., 266, 278
Kendrick, D. C., 228, 239
Kennard, J., 183, 197
Keys, A., 52, 54, 64
Khatami, M., 139, 145, 209, 220
Klein, D. F., 96, 111, 221, 266, 278, 279
Klerman, G. L., 114, 117, 125, 213, 222, 228, 231, 234, 239, 241
Kochansky, G. E., 156, 174
Koenig, H. G., 150, 155, 175
Kohlenberg, B. S., 164, 173
Koranyi, E. K., 94, 95, 96, 111
Koscis, J. H., 226, 227, 228, 236, 239, 266, 279

Kovaks, M., 141, 144
Kraepelin, E., 34, 47, 269, 279
Kraines, S. H., 227, 229, 230, 236, 240
Kronfol, T., 25, 29, 31
Krueger, Richard, 27, 31
Kubos, K. L., 39, 49
Kupfer, D. J., 209, 213, 219, 267, 269, 274, 275, 276, 279

L

LaRue, A., 154, 175
Lauritzen, L., 42, 46
Lawrence, P. S., 168, 174
Lawton, M. P., 150, 176
Leaf, P. H., 201, 222
Leaf, P. J., 69, 91
Leber, W. R., 219
Lee, S., 44, 49
Legh-Smith, J., 35, 49
Lestelle, V., 220, 221
Levenson, M. R., 148, 171
Levine, J. L., 141, 145
Levy, Elinor M., 27, 31
Levy, L. H., 86, 91
Lewin, L. M., 150, 162, 166, 175
Lewinsohn, P. M., 166, 172, 175
Lewis, A. B., 220, 221
Lewis, M., 83, 91
Liberman, Robert P., 203, 220
Lincoln, N. B., 35, 46
Linn, B. S., 88, 91
Linn, M. W., 88, 91
Lion, J. R., 124, 126
Lipkus, I. M., 89, 90
Lipman, R. S., 140, 143
Lipsey, J. R., 36, 39, 42, 47, 48
Litman, R., 120, 124, 126
Locke, S. E., 16, 31
London, W., 245, 248, 251, 252, 258, 262
Long, J. W., 246, 262
Lopez, J. F., 266, 277
Lovett, S., 166, 175
Lundervold, Duane A., 150, 162, 166, 175
Lustman, P. J., 209, 220
Lydiard, R. B., 108, 110

M

McCrainie, E. J., 184, 198
McCullough, J. P., 230, 233, 234, 240
McEachran, A. B., 219
McGarvey, B., 157, 175
McGlynn, E., 221

Pottash, A. C., 101, 111
Prendergast, D., 29, 31
Price, L. H., 278
Price, R. H., 202, 218
Price, T. R., 35, 38, 39, 41, 43, 46, 47, 48, 49
Prien, R. F., 267, 269, 272, 273, 274, 275, 276, 279
Prusoff, B. A., 206, 209, 213, 221, 222

Q

Quitkin, F., 111
Quitkin, F. M., 209, 213, 221

R

Rabin, A. S., 209, 221
Rabkin, J. G., 221
Rado, S., 182, 198
Rahe, R. H., 122, 126
Raphael, B., 38, 47
Rapp, S., 158, 176
Rasmussen, S. A., 278
Razzano, L., 219
Reding, M. J., 48
Rehm, L. P., 209, 215, 221
Reichlin, S., 28, 32
Rickels, K., 266, 279
Riddle, M. A., 209, 219
Rifkin, A., 111
Robinson, F. F., 88, 92
Robinson, L. A., 119, 126, 226, 235, 240
Robinson, Robert G., 35, 38, 39, 40, 41, 43, 45, 46, 47, 48, 49, 267, 276, 280
Rodman, J. L., 160, 176
Roffwarg, H. P., 209, 220
Rogers, W., 221, 222
Romano, J., 97, 112
Rose, T., 172
Roth, M., 34, 49
Rothschild, A. J., 25, 32
Rounsaville, B. J., 114, 125
Rovner, B. W., 176
Roy, L., 228, 240
Rozal, G. G., 69, 91
Ruegg, R. G., 149, 176
Rush, A. John, 128, 139, 140, 141, 142, 144, 145, 146, 220
Rush, A. J., 233, 234, 240

S

Sachar, E. J., 267, 280

Safran, J. D., 146
Salzinger, K., 166, 176
Samuels, J., 43, 47
Saul, L. J., 180, 198
Schaie, K. W., 67, 92
Schleifer, S., 26, 29, 32
Schmale, A., 3, 4, 13
Schmaling, K. B., 141, 144
Schneider, J., 160, 176
Schneider, P., 266, 278
Schooler, N., 206, 221
Schubert, D. S. P., 44, 49
Schulberg, H. C., 201, 219
Schultz, R., 149, 176
Schwab, J. J., 157, 176
Schwartz, D. A., 185, 194, 198
Schweizer, E., 266, 279
Schyler, D., 146
Scott, J., 227, 228, 231, 233, 234, 240, 241
Segal, Z. V., 146
Seligman, M. E. P., 83, 92
Sellers, D., 219
Shapiro, R. W., 94, 112
Shavit, Y., 24, 32
Shaw, B. F., 139, 140, 142, 145
Shea, M. T., 219
Shea, V., 44, 48
Sheik, J. I., 158, 177
Sherbourne, C. D., 205, 221
Shneidman, E. S., 120, 121, 126
Siegler, I. C., 89, 90
Simons, A. D., 141, 145, 209, 220
Sinyor, D., 35, 49
Skinner, B. F., 162, 163, 166, 177
Slagle, P., 263
Slawson, P.F., 185, 198
Smith, E., 17, 32
Smith, G., 263
Sotsky, S. M., 119, 126, 219
Spar, J. E., 154, 175
Spencer, J. H., 209, 215, 220, 221
Spiro, A. III, 148, 171
Spitz, R., 4, 13
Spitzer, R. L., 155, 172
Sprafkin, J. N., 150, 159, 173
Springer, C. J., 35, 41, 44, 46
Starkstein, S. E., 38, 39, 41, 46, 48, 49
Starr, L. B., 39, 49
Starvynski, A., 119, 126
Steffert, B., 184, 197
Stein, M., 32
Steinmetz, J., 157, 172
Steuer, J., 167, 177
Stewart, A., 201, 221, 222
Stewart, J. W., 209, 213, 221, 226, 241
Stiglin, L. E., 201, 220

Subject Index

A

of growing up, 192
of medications' side effects, 246
Feeling Good (Burns), 253
5-hydroxyindoleacetic acid (5-HIAA), 100
Fixation, at child level, 192
Fluoxetine (Prozac), 59, 272
Flushing, of upper body, 99
Fluvoxamine (Luvox), 272
Folate, 105
  deficiency, 106, 107
Fun, needed by depressed clients, 258
Functional wholeness, 116
Fusion, 190

G

G6 PDase deficiency, 108
General paresis, 106
Generations Together, 85
Geriatric depression
  See Depression, in older adults
Geriatric Depression Scale (GDS), 158
Gestalt therapy, 115
Glaucoma, 43
Glucocorticosteroids, 16, 17, 22
Granulocytes, 18
Gratification, autonomous, 185
Grief, 6-7, 122, 231
  acceptance of, 123
  cessation of medications for, 123
  resolution, 86
Group development
  phases of
    active phase, 80-81
    initial, 79-80
    termination phase, 81
Group therapy, 44, 115, 234
  curative influences of, 74, 76
  for depressed older adults, 65-90
  dynamics of elderly groups, 76-79
  for older white males, 72
  outpatient, 166-167
Groups
  assertiveness, 76
  elderly
    types of
      assertiveness training, 86-87
      bereavement, 86
      counseling and exercise, 87-89
      educational/therapeutic, 82-83
      intergenerational, 84-86

life review, 83-84
  psychodrama, 84
exercise, 76
gender selection, 78
inclusion of married and singles, 78
reminiscence, 83

H

Hallucinations, 142
Hallucinogenic drugs, 102
Hamilton Depression Rating Scale, 25, 26, 27, 42, 168, 169, 170, 204, 209, 216, 217
Health care team, 245
Health maintenance organization.
  See HMO
Heavy metal poisoning, 104
Helplessness, 83
Hepatitis, 105
Histamine, 99
HIV
  See Human immunodeficiency virus
HMO, 82, 83
Homework
  in cognitive therapy, 138-139
  for dysthymic patients, 234
Hope, remind clients of its existence, 247
Hopelessness, in dysthymic patients, 227
Hormones
  immune system and, 16
  neuroendocrine, 22
    depression and, 24-25
Hospice care, 122
Hospitalization, of depressed patient, 247
Hospitals, prevalence of depressed older adults in, 150
Hostels, elder, 82
Human immunodeficiency virus (HIV), 100
Humoral responses, 17
Huntington's Disease, 104-105
Hyperadrenalism (Cushing's Syndrome), 102
Hyperparathyroidism, 103-104
Hypertension, 88
Hypnotherapy, 115
Hypoadrenalism (Addison's Disease), 102-103
Hypoglycemia, 103

Contributors

Arnold E. Andersen, MD
Professor of Psychiatry, The University of Iowa College of Medicine, Iowa City, IA.

John A. Birtchnell, MD, FRC Psych., DPM, Dip. Psychother., AFBPsS
Honorary Senior Lecturer, the Institute of Psychiatry; Honorary Consultant Psychiatrist, the Maudsley Hospital, London, England.

Mary Ellen Copeland, MS
Counselor, Consultant, and Educator who specializes in the management of affective disorders and maintains a private practice in Brattleboro, VT.

Pedro L. Delgado, MD
Associate Professor of Psychiatry and Director of Psychopharmacology Research, University of Arizona College of Medicine, Tucson, AZ.

Cheryl Chancellor-Freeland, PhD
Immunology Fellow, Department of Microbiology, Boston University School of Medicine, Boston, MA.

Alan J. Gelenberg, MD
Professor and Head, Department of Psychiatry, University of Arizona College of Medicine, Tucson, AZ.

Shirley M. Glynn, PhD
Assistant Research Psychologist, Department of Psychiatry and Biobehavioral Sciences, UCLA School of Medicine, and Clinical Research Psychologist at the West Los Angeles Veterans Affairs Medical Center, Los Angeles, CA.

Mark S. Gold, MD
Potash Professor, University of Florida Brain Institute, Gainesville, FL.

Robert H. Howland, MD
Assistant Professor of Psychiatry, Western Psychiatric Institute and Clinic, University of Pittsburgh School of Medicine, Pittsburgh, PA.

Robin B. Jarrett, PhD
Associate Professor of Psychiatry, Department of Psychiatry, The
University of Texas Southwestern Medical Center, Dallas, TX.

Wanda Y. Johnson, PhD, PC
Licensed Professional Counselor, Licensed Marriage and Family
Therapist, Certified Hypnotherapist, and Certified Play Therapist in
private practice in Arlington, TX.

Richard Krueger, MD
Assistant Clinical Professor of Psychiatry, Columbia College of Physi-
cians and Surgeons, New York, NY; Attending Psychiatrist, Columbia
Presbyterian Hospital and the New York State Psychiatric Institute,
New York, NY.

Elinor M. Levy, PhD
Associate Professor of Microbiology, Department of Microbiology,
Boston University School of Medicine, Boston, MA.

Robert P. Liberman, MD
Professor, Department of Psychiatry and Biobehavioral Sciences, UCLA
School of Medicine; Director, Clinical Research Unit at Camarillo [CA]
State Hospital; Director, Clinical Research Center for the Study of
Schizophrenia; and Chief, Treatment Development and Assessment
Unit, Community and Rehabilitative Psychiatry Section, Psychiatry
Service, West Los Angeles Veterans Affairs Medical Center, Los Ange-
les, CA.

Duane A. Lundervold, RhD
Family Therapist, Boone County Youth and Family Counseling, Boone
County Hospital, Boone, IA.

Jim Mintz, PhD
Professor, Department of Psychiatry and Biobehavioral Sciences, UCLA
School of Medicine; Research Psychologist, West Los Angeles Veterans
Affairs Medical Center; and Chief, Methodology and Statistical Services
Unit, Clinical Research Center for the Study of Schizophrenia, Los
Angeles, CA.

Lois I. Mintz, PhD
Assistant Research Psychologist, Department of Psychiatry and Biobehavioral Sciences, UCLA School of Medicine, Los Angeles, CA.

Rajesh M. Parikh, MD
Associate Professor, Jaslok Hospital and Research Center, Bombay, India.

Mary Jane Robertson, MS
Research Associate, Department of Psychiatry and Biobehavioral Sciences, UCLA School of Medicine, Los Angeles, CA.

Robert G. Robinson, MD
Professor and Head, Department of Psychiatry, University of Iowa College of Medicine, Iowa City, IA.

A. John Rush, MD
Betty Jo Hay Professor of Psychiatry, Department of Psychiatry, The University of Texas Southwestern Medical Center, Dallas, TX.

Louis Jolyon West, MD
Professor of Psychiatry, UCLA School of Medicine, Los Angeles, CA.

Peter C. Whybrow, MD
Professor and Chairman, Department of Psychiatry, University of Pennsylvania, Philadelphia, PA.

For information on other books in
The Hatherleigh Guides series, call the
Marketing Department at Hatherleigh
Press, 1-800-367-2550, or write:
Hatherleigh Press
Marketing Department
420 E. 51st St.
New York, NY 10022